blind man's marathon

a journey through the third year of medical school

steven hatch

Printed in the United States of America.

Published by
WingSpan Press
Livermore, CA
www.wingspanpress.com

The WingSpan® name, logo and colophon are
the trademarks of WingSpan Publishing.

EAN 978-1-59594-038-4
ISBN 1-59594-038-3
First Edition 2006

Library of Congress Cataloging-in-Publication Data

Hatch, Steven.
   Blind man's marathon : a journey through the third year of
   medical school / Steven Hatch.-- 1st ed.
      p. cm.
   ISBN-13: 978-1-59594-038-4 (alk. paper)
   ISBN-10: 1-59594-038-3 (alk. paper)
1. Hatch, Steven. 2. Medical students--United States--
Biography. 3. Medicine--Study and teaching--United States.
I. Title.
   R745.H42 2005
   610.71'173--dc22

                              2005034020

for Miriam

acknowledgements

I'd like to thank the following people for their help in producing this book: Mark Meyers did some serious low-cost (i.e. free) copy editing of seemingly endless revisions and his enthusiasm for my writing never waned. Natalie DeNormandie, ever the artist, conceived of a cover that neatly illustrates exactly what it felt like to be a student as you hit the wards — perhaps demonstrating that a picture can be worth 100,000 words. My parents, Herb and Lee Hatch, as well as my in-laws, Murray and Helene Tuchman, all provided feedback that helped to weed out the more tangential material.

A few classmates from Cincinnati, especially Allison Oppenheimer, Scott Pentiuk, Michael Tuchfarber, Aaron Boster and Himansh Khana, also cheered me on while I was trying to be a top-flight student (during most of my rotations, at any rate) and simultaneously keep the journal that formed the core of this book. These guys have all made me a better person, and, I hope, a better doctor.

Rick Kopelman, my residency director, graciously helped us with the front-cover photo shoot. Besides that, he was unwavering in his support of me during my internship while I was trying to balance raising twins and figure out how to learn medicine, a task which I found out was much more difficult than I could have ever predicted. I do not think I would have made it through the year without his gentle encouragement. If you are interested in an internal medicine residency in Boston, the reason to come to Tufts is because Rick is there.

The contributions of all these people, substantial though they are, pall in comparison to those of my wife, Miriam, who has fiercely maintained a belief that this book should be published and "has something to say," even when I have felt overly discouraged and wanted to quit. I am phenomenally lucky to have a partner who believes in what I do.

author's note

This book represents a factual account of my experiences during my third year of medical school in Cincinnati, Ohio. However, in the interests of patient privacy, I have deliberately changed all names and details regarding their lives (their residences, jobs, the color of their hair, any unusual physical characteristics, among many other things) such that no patient or family member should be able to recognize themselves — or fear that their lives are being exposed — in the following pages. The faculty, staff, and residents from the various hospitals where I worked, as well as my classmates, have also had their names changed. Aside from me and my wife, the only person whose real name is in this book is that of Dr. Jeanne Ballard, a renowned neonatologist at Children's Hospital whom I mention in passing for reasons which are clear in the chapter on pediatrics.

On a separate note involving shameless self-promotion: this book is being self-published using internet and small-print technology, and as such any chance it has of being successful will require word-of-mouth and the willingness of people to purchase the book from internet websites such as overlookedbooks.com or amazon.com. Thus, if you enjoy the read, I humbly ask that you spread the word to friends and colleagues and direct them to the above websites.

Waltham, Mass.
2005

introduction

starting in the middle:

the day before the boards

Thursday, June 15

Twenty four hours from now, I will get up from a small cubicle with a computer, walk out of the Test Center where I will have been sitting all day, and I will end, at least symbolically, my second year of medical school. In reality, the academic school year ended five weeks ago, in early May, when we took the last final exam of the spring quarter on Pathology, truly a hellacious experience in which a passing grade was awarded for correctly answering only one out of every two questions asked. At that point, those students left standing had finished the second-year requirements.

But in order to begin the third year, medical students must take and pass the United States Medical Licensing Examination, Step One. The USMLE exams are part of a three-tiered process through which all aspiring doctors must pass during medical school and the early years of residency. Step One attempts to measure a student's proficiency in the "basic sciences" taught during the first two years, subjects such as biochemistry, gross anatomy, histology, pathology, microbiology, and the like. Sometimes students refer to the tests by their "Step" names (Step One, Step Two, Step Three), but mostly everyone calls them *the boards*, perhaps because the term "step" implies ascendancy, whereas the term "board" sounds like an implement that can thwack one on the head.

In previous years, nearly all medical students in the United States took the boards on the same day in early June, right before the start of the third year. Now, however, students may take the test anytime before the third year begins in July. Some classmates of mine have chosen to study only two weeks for the boards, while others have given themselves the maximum six weeks. I wanted to take a vacation before third year started, so I've allotted four weeks to study and am taking the test tomorrow. Clearly, I'm making the most of my final hours.

I mean, I *could* sit at my library table, books stacked three high, from now until midnight, trying to put into short-term memory all the facts that I think might be asked of me tomorrow.

3

But I figure it this way. There's 350 questions on the exam. One third of the questions will be easy, one third will be possible to answer if I concentrate, and the final third I won't be able to get no matter how hard I study. Thus, I'm here typing instead of knocking myself out. As the weeks have gone by I've been fairly disheartened as I watched the parade of students finished with the boards come marching—indeed, skipping—through the library, ecstatic that they're finally free, while I had to continue on looking over my notes for the *nth* time: *the glycolytic pathway begins with glucose, which is converted to glucose-6-phosphate, and then converted to fructose-6-phosphate....*

Maybe I'm rationalizing, though. I *always* take my foot off the gas pedal before exams. It's my way of coping with the stress. And it's very easy to get stressed when you take exams in medical school. Except for extremely talented students, there are simply too many facts to keep straight. It's probably harder to cope with the *realization* of how much you're expected to learn rather than the learning itself. You'll look at your calendar two weeks out from a test and think, "Wait, I have fourteen days to learn all *that?*"

And when you get to that point, unless you can keep your wits about you, you'll either Go Off The Deep End, spending every possible minute studying, getting upset with your body when it addresses its own selfish needs such as eating, sleeping, and defecating, or you'll simply give up, thinking it can't be done. If you approach your studies either way for any sustained period of time, you run a high risk of buying an early ticket out of med school.

One fellow student, Bob Beatty, was squarely in the former group. He was very serious about doing the absolute best he could in school. He didn't want to merely pass; he wanted to be in the top twenty percent—an honors student. Such students are destined to be in the national honors society of medicine: Alpha Omega Alpha, or simply "AOA." On one level I respected that, understanding that he was dedicated to working as hard as he could to achieve his goals, and like the slogan in the Army, he wanted to be all that he could be. But often Bob would carry this zeal to excess, remaining at the medical school for days on end, studying through the night, falling asleep at 6 a.m., then waking up exhausted at nine or ten and dragging himself to lecture, where he tended to fall asleep. Or he would drink enough coffee to stay awake, furiously scribbling notes. After awhile, and especially during the week before exams, the strain was clearly evident on his face. Even a light tap on his shoulder to say 'good morning' could cause a dramatic startle response—"WHAT! WHAT DO YOU WANT!! OH! I'M FINE!" In order to avoid the complications of laundry, he would wear operating room clothes provided by the hospital. After a few weeks of wearing such apparel, some fellow classmates wryly dubbed him "Scrub."

Those students who gave up washed out of med school a long time ago, mostly during the first few weeks. We probably lost five or six out of 165 that way, and I have no doubt that their aptitude had little to do with their departure. Either they realized that medicine wasn't what they *really* wanted to do and that it was Daddy's dream all along, or that they simply froze up when they were hit with the first onslaught of information. Succeeding in medical school—in the first two years, at any rate, when your social skills aren't called upon—doesn't require stunning intelligence. It requires a determination to stare at a book as long as you can to remember as much as is humanly possible, and the presence of mind to not be intimidated by all that you are required to learn.

Obviously a good memory helps. I'm not sure if genuine creativity and intelligence helps or hinders you, since so much of the first two years is based on rote memorization, which can be mind-numbing for truly creative people. I've concluded that dogged determination is probably a better predictor of where you'll land in the class standings than any other variable. The question you must ask yourself, as a medical student, is this: do I want to study *four* hours a day to learn the material in a basic outline, do I want to study *six* hours a day to learn the material in a more detailed fashion, or do I want to study *eight* or more hours each day to know each subject cold?

Although I would very much like to be at the top of the class and would like to possess that dogged determination, I'm somewhere in the ballpark of the "six hours a day" group, and my class standing is pretty much in the middle of the pack after two years. I'm not going to end up being a brain surgeon. Shucks. Which brings us back to the USMLE Step One, arguably the most important exam that all medical students take, and the sad but true fact that I have been taking it *easier* as I've come closer to the exam and not pouring it on.

α α α α α α α α α

Why would I begin telling you a story at the *halfway* point in medical school?

In reality, medical school is two separate experiences divided into blocks of two years each. The first part is mostly "academic," where the vast majority of time is spent in the relatively sterile confines of the classroom and the library (or study spot of choice). You only spend a little bit of time working with actual physicians, learning the basics of physical diagnosis and just getting a feel for life in the hospital or the doctor's office. But the first two years aren't much different from the undergraduate premedical classes that are required to enter medical school. Your aptitude is still measured exclusively by taking tests, which most of the time consists of filling in little bubbles on Scan-tron sheets, choosing from one of four or five answers to a question.

Some schools take slightly different approaches to how they teach the first two years. Still, as a rule, most medical schools teach the basics during the first two years by telling their students to plant their asses in front of books and *start memorizing!*

By contrast, the third year is the *real* beginning of medical school. It's the first period where students spend substantial time interacting directly with patients, where *gastric carcinoma* is no longer a bunch of information on a page but rather a person lying in a hospital bed looking to you and the rest of the medical staff for help. Third year is the time when smarts won't guide you through every narrow passage. To do well in third year requires what is needed in all good physicians:

6

compassion, gentleness, and a social intangible that I think of as simply *the touch*. It's the ability to make a connection with people—not just the patients and their families, but other physicians, the nursing staff, the orderlies, everyone.

Book smarts are still quite important, as the third-year course grades are still determined in part by "objective" tests. But because the "subjective" evaluation-based grades prize qualities very different from those rewarded during the first two years, many students undergo a flip-flop in class standing. Some students that had not been especially successful during the basic science years can make meteoric rises in class rank, while others that have always excelled in academics but never been required to utilize subtle social skills can find themselves dropping like rocks. Or so the rumors go, anyway.

A third year student is the lowest person on the medical ladder in a profession that's extremely hierarchical, and that ladder includes more than just other doctors. *Everyone* can pull rank on a third year, since even the IV therapist has more patient experience and works everyday with the rest of the medical staff. A third year, by contrast, is just a passerby, and will be gone by the end of the month. Even the slightest whiff of arrogance or nastiness can spell disaster, because if you don't work well with the staff or the patients, the word about you will travel fast.

Because the third year is the one in which students are called upon to learn and display the skills that are normally required of doctors, having good grades during the third year is of critical importance. At the University of Cincinnati, third year grades are worth the equivalent of the first two years combined; many other schools only have pass-fail grades during the first two years, and don't start tallying class rank until the third year.

If this seems anxiety provoking, the method of grading during the third year adds yet more adrenaline to the pot, because students are judged *directly* against other classmates. That is, a passing performance is considered to be one *expected* of a third year student. The higher grades—high passes and honors—are reserved for those students who are considered by the course directors to be a cut above other students. This sounds reasonable, and indeed it is.

Still, try explaining *that* to a student who has gotten lots of A's and a few B's for the past sixteen, seventeen years. When a 3.8 lifetime student drops down to a 2.6 GPA halfway through medical school, there's hell to pay somewhere. When I've sat around in the student lounge, eating lunch, I've chatted with the current third-but-soon-to-be-fourth years, and to say that they complain bitterly doesn't adequately give you a sense of the acidity of their feelings.

We'll see how I tolerate third-year evaluations. I have an advantage in that I was *never* a top-flight student, much more content to be a lazy bottom-feeder and just get by with what natural smarts I had. But we'll save that topic for a later date.

Third year grades are so important, incidentally, not least because they dictate your choice of medical subspecialty. The higher your class standing (which means lots of "honors" during your third year), the more options you have of choosing what you want to pursue and where you want to pursue it. Some of the more competitive residencies such as dermatology, radiology, and urology — specialties which have the advantages of light call, handsome incomes, fairly regular working hours, and frequently healthy patients — often look only at top-ranked students. So if you've done well during your first two years and you want to be a radiologist, it's critical that you continue to pull down top grades, or else it might be time to consider another specialty, which can be a traumatic event if you've spent two years banking on that cushy radiology job.

On the upside, third year is also a time when you, as a student, get to sample from the smorgasbord of medicine. You're not constrained by the perspective of only one specialty, although eventually everyone goes down the path of specializing. The third year's when you get to try on the clothes of a psychiatrist even if you know that you don't want to do psychiatry; when you get to play surgeon although you have no intention of seeing the inside of an operating room again until you yourself are under the knife; when some (foolish) parent will hand you their six month-old baby, *willingly*, and ask you to stick an otoscope in the baby's ear to lock for an infection.

It's the only year in your professional life when you get to be every kind of doctor and savor each taste separately. From all I've heard, the candy-store like atmosphere of the third year can take people who were certain that they wanted to be general surgeons and make them wonder why they'd want to do anything other than pediatrics, or make people who thought they'd want to do radiology realize that there's no way they're going to spend their entire professional lives in the dimly lit bowels of a hospital. Some students will come to the end of third year not knowing what they want to do because they liked everything, and some students will come to the end of third year not knowing what they want to do because they didn't like *anything*.

If one is to succeed throughout this year while running the gauntlet of all these different specialties, each with their own culture and language, one must possess stamina and maintain focus. Medical school, especially the third year, is a marathon, not a sprint. The catch to this marathon is that your ignorance is so profound you run it as a blind man would, unable to appreciate the twists and turns in the road until you've already veered off the path and fallen flat on your face.

α α α α α α α α α

With all these factors at play during the course of twelve months, there's no question in my mind that the third year is the most pivotal year not only of medical school, but of a physician's career. The third year marks the period when a person who thinks like a medical student turns into one who thinks like a doctor, and the two are very different things. Pre-clinical medical students are good at thinking about separate subjects. They can tell you a lot about the different flavors of *Salmonella* infection and the functions of the different interleukin molecules secreted by white blood cells. What they can't do is evaluate a patient who comes in saying, "Well, I hurt right *here*."

To my knowledge, there is at least one well-known book written about the first year of medical school, an account of the first year at Harvard Medical School by Charles LeBaron called *Gentle Vengeance*. Many books have been written about the intern experience, the most famous being the minor classic of American literature *The House of God* by Samuel Shem. There are a few other accounts about the entire medical school experience, including Perri Klass's memoir *A Not Entirely Benign Procedure*. There's even a book written about just *one course* in med school — gross anatomy, which claims it's the most important course in a physician's education. (Silly author: *any* medical student could tell you that the most important courses during the basic science years are pathology and physiology.)

Yet I've never heard of an account focusing solely on the all-important third year, and that's why I'm writing this book. Maybe there's one out there, but oh well, guess I should've researched the book market more thoroughly in my spare time.

I also don't know of any student accounts from those who attend schools that aren't called "Harvard." Given that there's about 120 medical schools in the US, that's a skewed perspective. There's a whole mess of schools out there that are composed of very talented students who didn't attend Ivy League schools or didn't get 3.9 GPAs in college (they averaged, say, 3.6 instead) — public Universities which often have the surname *State* (Ohio State, Penn State) and don't inspire the same awe as schools with a handsome pedigree. That's where the majority of students go to medical school, though, and the perspective from the corn fields of the Midwest might be different than that from Mount Harvard.

Not that I have anything against Harvard and schools of its ilk — University of Chicago, Cornell, UCSF, Columbia and whatnot. Nevertheless, this book seeks to talk about the *average* experience of a third year medical student, and what better place to do that than at a medical school that is ranked, according to US News and World Report, 46th out of 120 schools?

It's important because the concerns of average medical students at average medical schools are tied directly to the strength of their schools' reputations. Even sub-par students from Johns Hopkins are likely to have an easier time of it applying to competitive residencies than slightly-above-average students at University of Cincinnati. If you want to get into a good residency, that's the uphill battle you have to fight.

Obviously I'm writing about my own experiences, and although I try to talk a good game about the "average medical student," at thirty years old, and with a Master's degree in English Literature under my belt, I'm not exactly the poster child for Conventional Medical Student. Still, I believe that most medical students experience similar ups and downs, are subject to similar forms of hazing and praise, and share the same frustrations and satisfactions as the year progresses. Not every student shares my preoccupations with grades, my insecurities, and my strengths. I can't write Everyman's account, but I can write with honesty about my own experiences, and in doing so paint a portrait of this critical year in a physician's professional life.

When in doubt, cut it out.
— Brad Crafton, MD

<u>one</u>

cutting it up with the general surgeons

Saturday, July 1

Our two-day orientation to third year is behind us, we have the weekend off, and we charge boldly into the fray on Monday. The basic gist of the orientation was "how not to make a complete fuck-up of yourself next year" and, if indeed that was the goal of the orientation committee, they got the point across successfully, which is good, since I'm jumping into the deep end for my first rotation. I'm in Surgery.

As surgery goes, I'm relatively lucky. We have to do two one-month rotations in various hospitals, and my two hospitals are generally considered benign—the Christ Hospital and the Veteran's Administration, or VA, Hospital. When I got the request list for which rotations were available, I headed directly to a third-year and asked her what was different about the rotations. "Just make sure you don't request University Team One," she said with the same kind of tone that parents use when they tell their children not to stick their fingers in light sockets.

University Hospital Surgery Team One has a notorious reputation. Students talk about Team One the same way people talk about going through basic training in the army. The surgeons are mean-spirited and observe a strict hierarchy with the implicit assumption that the word "hierarchy" means the right to treat the person on the rung below as cruelly as they see fit. They thrive on intimidation and humiliation. I heard a story that a Team One surgeon was once asking a student some arcane anatomy question, and when the student couldn't answer, the surgeon flung the scalpel he was using toward the student in disgust.* I talked to another student who said he had been kept up two consecutive nights to observe surgeries and was relentlessly questioned by the attendings. He finally had had enough, told his superiors that he wasn't

---

* I later learned from the Surgery course director that the story was true. After the surgeon had flung the scalpel at the student, word had gotten out to his colleagues of the incident. When confronted, he expressed indifference. "But you could have *hurt* the boy!" a fellow surgeon chided. "Oh no," he replied, "If I had meant to hurt him, I would not have *missed*."

gaining from the experience, and walked out of the OR and went home to sleep—after staying awake for more than 40 consecutive hours.

These stories may be embellished, but the sheer volume of horror stories I hear suggest to me that Team One is either filled with a nasty bunch of critters, or they need to hire a new public relations firm and quick. I have no desire to be anywhere near that kind of a learning experience, so I requested the Christ Hospital and the VA at the top of my list, and all the University rotations at the bottom. Not long after I submitted my requests I ran into a fellow student who remarked that she had put all her Team One requests in the middle. "The middle?" I asked. "Why the middle?"

"Because if they see you putting their rotations all at the bottom, they'll automatically assign you Team One," she said knowingly.

I thought my bowels were going to evacuate at that moment.

Obviously this turned out not to be true. The Christ and VA rotations are considered downright cushy compared to the University experience. Our call schedule is every fourth night—same as the University—but our non-call schedule is only about 6:00 a.m. to 5:00 or 6:00 p.m. Team One can start at 4:30 a.m. and run until 9:00 at night. Mind you, this is the easy part of the schedule—a call night day will start at the same early hour, go straight through the night, and continue all the way until 9:00 the following evening. Then, after possibly 41 hours of consecutive work, you drive home to get a maximum of seven hours of sleep, because you're back on duty at 4:30!

The residents work on schedules like this for up to five years, until they're finally full-blown surgeons. Clearly, to survive this kind of hellish experience one has got to have an iron will and an absolute sense of determination. I can appreciate that in the same way that I appreciate the dedication of professional athletes, but I don't understand it at all. I also can't grasp how anyone thinks that it's safe for someone to be evaluating patients, prescribing medicines, and of all things *performing surgeries*, on that little an amount of sleep. Federal and state governments have considerably more strict requirements on heavy machine operators or truck drivers.

Wednesday, July 5

I couldn't get to sleep last night, so instead of being well rested, ready to hit the ground running at 5:00 a.m., I was out of bed by 4:30 and at the hospital an hour later. It turned out not to do a lot of good to be there so early. None of the residents were in sight until 6:00, so I ambled about the very dead hospital for the half-hour, trying to figure out where to put my books, since I had not yet figured out where my locker was.

At 6:00 a.m. we had morning rounds, a quick check-up on the patients who had undergone operations. Four residents checked about 15 or so patients in just over an hour. It didn't seem like a very organized affair. The residents apparently randomly went after patients, and if one of the residents was already checking out that patient, they checked it off their list and moved on to the next. It seemed to me to follow the principles of a golf scramble: Start your work after the person who went the farthest. During this time, my classmate Jason Vincent and I followed around whichever resident was nearest, not really knowing what to do or say or ask.

By 7:30, we were due a mile away at the University Hospital for Grand Rounds, so we packed into our cars and drove over. Grand Rounds is a once-a-week affair done in all hospital departments, and consists of a lecture or lectures designed to keep students, residents, and attendings up to date on the latest advances in basic science or clinical medicine. I can tell you this: The first lecture had something to do with a protein called "IL-6," and the second lecture described research on male rats. I can't tell you much beyond that. My guess is that I took more away from those talks than about half of the students and residents there. It's simply too hard to focus the mind that early in the morning, especially if one is sleep deprived, and a resident fits that bill.

Back at the Christ by 9:00 am and I'm scrubbing in on my first surgery with Dr. Blaston, an exploratory surgery to look for complications in a woman who had had a "Whipple" procedure performed last year, a very complicated surgery for patients with pancreatic cancer. He's an imposing man by any standard since he stands about six foot seven, but more importantly, he has the knack of being able to let you know he is scowling at you despite his face being hidden behind his surgical mask.

The chief resident, Scott Gleason, gestured to me to scrub by him at the sink, and quietly explained that the first rule to learn is *never* to scrub in before the attending unless explicitly instructed otherwise and *never* to finish scrubbing before anyone. When I come in, Blaston and Gleason have already cut the patient open and are chatting as they work. I'm standing there, arms wet, held out in the air so as not to touch anything. The scrub nurse hands me a towel, which I use to dry off my hands very carefully to maintain a sterile environment. The scrub nurse gestures to come over to her so that she may gown me, and asks if I'm new. I say yes, this is my first day of my third year. She rolls her eyes with an *oh boy* look. Finally suited up, I wait for instructions as to where to stand, which turns out to be next to Blaston.

"Okay doc. What's the survival rate for a patient with pancreatic mets?"

"Pimping" is the time-honored tradition among physicians and their students whereby the physician ostensibly teaches a student and simultaneously evaluates his or her fund of medical knowledge. In theory, the doctor will ask a student a question about some medical topic, and the prepared student will respond with the correct answer, at which point the doctor will proceed to expand on the chosen topic or keep asking questions until the student runs out of answers.

I guessed, knowing I was in the ballpark: "Five..."

"Zero!" came the swift response. "Median survival of nine to twelve months." His tone was of utter disdain. "What's the typical presenting clinical symptom of pancreatic cancer?"

I was stumped, and I knew I shouldn't have been. "Acute pancreatitis?" I ventured.

"Almost never."

I stood there. About thirty seconds passed.

"We're *waiting*...." with the same voice tones as Jack Nicholson saying "Here's *Johnny!*"

"I'm sorry, doctor? Did you ask for an instrument?" the surprised nurse asked.

"No, he's waiting for me," I boldly and stupidly offered. "Fat malabsorption and steatorrhea?" This was almost as whacked a guess as the first but it seemed like a gamer.

Exasperation. "Doc, you're going to need to *think* about the disease to arrive at the answer. *Think* about it."

One of the nurses clucked, "Doctor Blaston, you're being tough on the student today! His first day!"

"Him? Oh, he's just a *turd.*"

Silence again. Back under my shell I went. Mind you, the surgery was hardly a den of solemnity until The Pimping. Blaston was chirping back and forth with his anesthetist and nurses. He was slightly abrasive with the chief resident—*Scott, cut there! No, don't pull that tight!* Dave Matthews was playing quietly from the boom box five feet away.

About thirty minutes later my brain finally started to function in the way it had functioned a few months ago. Pancreatic tumors are mostly in the head of the pancreas, which is where the bile duct empties into the duodenum, the beginning of the small intestine. A tumor there is going to block up the duct, and all that bile's gonna get backed up. "Doctor, may I ask a question?"

"Mmmm."

"Is it cholestasis?" Fancy word simply meaning backup of bile.

"No, but *now* you're thinking on the right track." Looking right at me now. "Take it one step further." Tone neither encouraging nor discouraging, just matter of fact.

"....um, jaundice?"

"That's right. Painless jaundice is a *very* bad sign. And I want you to find out what Curvoisier's sign is and why that's important."

This entire exchange followed the thoroughly depressing

news that the samples we had sent to surgical pathology came back as positive for pancreatic metastatic cancer. I had met the woman only hours before. My first case and she's not going to live through this journal. It's an unhappy, sobering thought, but the team was not weepy through the rest of the surgery (which lasted three hours total, and we found out about the recurrent cancer at the end of the first hour). The atmosphere was a bit more subdued, but business went on as usual.

Surgery over and out by 12:00, followed by a drug rep lunch. Drug rep lunches are the most common way overworked residents and interns get their nutrition, and the residents greet these events with almost gleeful anticipation. These lunches function, effectively, as high-priced commercials: A sales representative from a drug company will come in and tout their product—say, "Dipstrix" medication for chronic stupidity—giving a five-minute shpiel about how marvelous a drug it is. While they drone on about the elixir-like properties of their medication, the physicians chomp away at little deli boxes that contain very nice chicken-salad croissant sandwiches with a little pasta salad, a piece of fruit, a can of pop, and a cookie. Everyone swears this has no effect on their prescription patterns. I believe that about as much as I believe that teenagers aren't influenced by beer and cigarette advertisements.

Clinic at 1:00. I saw a patient with cellulitis, an infection of soft tissue, and didn't know what I was doing. I mean, I vaguely know how to take a cursory history and perform a minimally competent physical, but I don't know what the surgery people want me to look for. I think it's going to be weeks of this before I even begin to have a clue.

Back in the car, over to the University for the 2:00 lecture. We got there at 2:25. It was on abdominal surgery—just a general think-through about what basic issues should be going through your head when you see patients with abdominal pain. The hardest part of medical school, I think right now, is keeping all the damn information *straight*. You'll learn about all the presenting signs and symptoms of pancreatitis, for instance, and you'll think, okay, I've got it *down* and wrapped up. Nailed that information to my brain. Then, a few days later, you have to learn about, say, hepatitis, and you think, wait a minute, doesn't that sound a little bit like something that I remember reading about pancreatitis? Or the stomach. Or the small intestine. Or some bug from South America that you're guaranteed never to see in your career but still you memorized it because *it was on the test*. And you realize that you spent a lot of hours in the library and you're not sure if any good came of it.

Saturday, July 8

It took three full days, but I know now that I have no desire to be a surgeon. I probably could have told you that three days ago, but it's good to keep an open mind about these things.

Not that I haven't been having fun sitting in on the surgeries. When I'm not worried about contaminating myself in the OR or making sure I'm holding the retractor just so, I take a moment to think *wow, wow, wow*. There we are, probing around inside the stomach of a woman who has just been effectively disemboweled, her guts are being tossed to and fro, and in a few short hours she's going to be completely sewn back up again. That's amazing.

Not that the OR is a place where people are busy thinking or saying *wow wow wow*. Once the patient is under anesthesia the OR turns into a mechanic's workshop, only cleaner. The atmosphere is generally casual — well, maybe "casual" isn't the right word. I don't want to give the impression that as soon as the patient goes under, the staff starts partying. But the kind of nail-biting tension that the family feels in the waiting room is nowhere to be found in the OR suite. The staff simply couldn't maintain that kind of intensity if they felt that way for every case that came through.

I *did* have a fun moment when I was sitting in with a plastic surgeon who was reconstructing a breast that had just been removed by the general surgery team. The boom box was playing fairly loudly, and the surgeon decided it was time to pimp me.

"Doctor Hatch."

"Yes, doctor?"

21

"Name the song that's playing."

"That would be *Bohemian Rhapsody*, by Queen, doctor."

"You're doing very well, Doctor Hatch."

$$$$$$$

Yesterday I was in surgery doing a mastectomy with Dr. Silverman, the attending who writes my grade. This is my first time meeting him, and first impressions are going to mean a lot. I studied breast cancer the night before, so I felt reasonably confident in answering at least some of his questions. Assisting him was Armand, who's in his second year of residency. That means that he's almost as low on the totem pole as me. It means he's likely going to get hammered by the attending, perhaps even worse than me since he's in the club—of surgeons, that is. We're ten or twenty minutes into the surgery and Armand's tentativeness was entirely apparent. He didn't have much practice with mastectomies and Silverman was fairly stern with him, but not abusive. (I didn't know it at the time, but Armand apparently was on Silverman's bad side for some kind of misunderstanding that arose last year. Armand was talking to a patient's family, and I don't know the details but he clearly said something that made Silverman look bad.)

"*No*...don't cut so deep," Silverman said. "And don't be so tentative. It's only a breast. Steven, how do you diagnose breast cancer?"

Fortunately he started me out with an easy one. "Masses larger than one centimeter can be found on palpation either by self-exam or in the office. Otherwise they can be picked up on mammography or ultrasound screening."

"Very good. What are the recommendations for screening?"

My moment to impress had arrived. "Do you want the IOM recommendations or the American Cancer Society's?"

Dr. Silverman stopped, looked up and laughed at me. The nurse anesthetist said, "Hey, I want this guy to operate on me!"

"Feel free to tell me either," Silverman said. I told him both. Chance to score on another front. "My residents have been teaching me well."

"Ah-ah-ah, Doctor Hatch," Silverman quickly cut in. "There's a skill to this, Steven. You suck up to *me*, not him."

"Fair enough," I said. He was not only right, the line sounded pretty stupid anyway. It smacked of the kind of craven bootlicking that I was determined never to do.

The biggest surprise of that morning was hearing Silverman say it's *only* a breast. I have absolutely no doubt that he was talking as a surgeon to a tentative surgical resident, trying to reassure him in order to get him to move more swiftly and confidently. When you operate on the stomach, there's a whole mess of structures that you *don't* want to cut or even come near. Not so with much of the breast, which is "simply" a modified sweat gland that is well separated from any major arteries and all but two major nerves. Still, I wondered if the female nurses and techs in the room didn't get a chill when he delivered that zinger. He may not have literally meant that this was just another woman or just another piece of female flesh on the table, but still, given medicine's track record with women, it was a brassy observation.

Tuesday, July 11   post-call

On Monday I was trying to kill an hour before going to the outpatient clinic, and I saw that Dr. Caffey was doing a minor procedure for a man with hemorrhoids. This was not a "surgery" proper, as no cutting was involved. I thought it sounded somewhat boring but figured it would pass the time. I bumped into Caffey in the hallway and introduced myself. "Hi Dr. Caffey," I said. "I was wondering if it was okay to sit in on your next case."

"Sure, that's fine. And you are....."

"Steven Hatch, UC three," denoting my position on the food chain.

The patient was placed prone (on his stomach) on the operating table, and he was given a drug called *propofol* to sedate him. Propofol is a great sedative, but it has the sometimes undesirable effect of causing respiratory depression. Usually this is mild and can be controlled by both an alert anesthetist and an endotracheal tube which can deliver oxygen to the lungs even if the patient doesn't make a good attempt to breathe. But because of this side effect, some doctors prefer mixing propofol with a drug called *ketamine*. Ketamine will act as a physiological *stimulant*, which counteracts the respiratory depression-inducing effect of propofol. The drawback is that patients can hallucinate, and may become combative and violent. This anesthetist wasn't going to use ketamine.

I expected only to establish good rapport with the patient and practice my bedside skills a bit and do nothing else. Once we had transferred the patient from his bed to the table, I began to move the bed out of the OR, as I had seen done on the half-dozen other operations that I sat in on. "Hold it, don't take that bed anywhere," was Caffey's firm but unexplained response. I moved it off to the side.

About a minute into the procedure the nurse anesthetist very quickly said, "He's down to seventy over fifty," and from that moment for about the next, say, forty-five seconds, everything was a whir to me. I remember Caffey say coolly, "We've got to get him flipped over," then repeat it with more intensity, then repeat it with even greater intensity and volume but not to the point of yelling. I remember the anesthetist moving wildly about the head of the patient, yelping, "he's turning purple!"

I was just standing there, but immediately I was summoned to get the very bed that I had wanted to move out of the room. I did so, and took a crash-course in applying the "bed-brakes" to stabilize the bed for transferring the patient, which I was ordered to do with haste. While I was doing this, the OR nurse tried to manipulate the OR table, which had been lowered and specially adjusted for the procedure. She was trying to raise and flatten the bed by the control box attached to the table motor, but she wasn't getting it to work properly. Then my resident Shelly stepped in. Maybe fifteen seconds have passed now. She can't get the thing to work. Caffey is now at her most intense—

still firmly in control, but the urgency of the situation is now obvious to all of us — she's saying that he *must* get flipped *now* and that means that that bed needs to be up *now*.

Five or so seconds elapse, and Caffey is now working the controls, and like magic, the table is rising. The patient is truly purple. Finally the table is level with the bed and the patient is ready to be rolled. I am the only male in the room, there are four relatively small women, and *I'm* the one who's on the far side of the bed, the farthest away from the patient. Shelly now takes Caffey's tone with me and says that *it's time to move him and we need you to help. Now, Steven!* One "don't be shy" later from Caffey and I'm putting my bulk into it, and as we pass the half-minute mark the man is now lying on his back, off the anesthesia, and taking oxygen. We get him stabilized over the next minute or two, roll him back onto the table (he's groggy, kind-of half-awake since we got him back onto his bed, but he'll certainly not remember the experience — yet another side effect of the propofol), and once we re-sterilize ourselves, he's gone under again, and we're back to work as if nothing at all happened.

But it didn't take a genius to see that Caffey was livid. Later when we were out of the OR (procedure successful), I approached her and asked what had just happened. She gave me the run-down on ketamine and propofol (and her own strongly held opinion that ketamine was clearly indicated in this instance). I tried to be a bit glib, and expressed surprise that I had to sit in on a hemorrhoid operation to see the most exciting surgery of my clerkship.

Aside from me, these were all very experienced professionals in the OR performing a fairly simple and routine procedure. But it provided a window as to what happens when a problem develops and is compounded by other mistakes — the table can't be adjusted properly by the personnel, the bed isn't in the room, someone loses their cool. Of these things, the table eventually *was* adjusted, the bed thankfully *was* in the room (only because of Caffey's insistence; another, less stringent doctor might have let it slide by), and save the nurse anesthetist, everyone else was generally calm. But those were all near-misses; any one of those elements change and a patient who came in for hemorrhoids could have left much worse, or not left at all. I think the only reason why things didn't completely disintegrate was because of Caffey, who directed us all like a general directs the troops in the heat of battle. A general that wins, that is.

Then today I was talking to my resident Armand. Since we were both on call the night before (I got about four hours of sleep, a good deal more than he did), we were talking about what it's like to work tired, and he was sharing some stories with me about how tired he has been when taking call on such little sleep. I asked him if any mistakes had occurred as a result.

"You know, this one time, when I was an intern, I had this patient whose platelets were getting pretty low in the middle of the night, like down to 80 or 40 or something," he said. Platelet counts should be at least 250 (thousand), so a count between 40 and 80 is a cause for genuine concern. "I paged the resident, and I don't think he was fully awake when he was talking to me, and I explained the situation to him and he said, 'No, no, don't worry about it, let's take another platelet count in the morning and see how he's doing then.' That didn't sound good to me but what did I know, you know? I was just an intern and he was a resident. I'm not even sure he woke up enough to remember the call. By the next morning the guy's platelets were at, like, eight. The guy didn't make it. I'm not sure he would have anyway, but that didn't help much."

So only five full days of surgery and I'm becoming even more convinced that this call stuff is not just stupid in terms of making residents feel constantly tired and run-down, but that it literally can put patients' lives in danger. I don't know about you, but if it were my hemorrhoid operation and my blood pressure went south, I wouldn't want an exhausted resident searching around for how to lift up the table while I slowly choked to death.

Above all things, avoid any ridiculous expressions of humour, at the bed-side of a sick man; you cannot choose a more unseasonable opportunity for your Mirth.
— **Samuel Bard, MD, 1769**

My one exciting moment during call last night came at the end of what at the time seemed like a very satisfying dream, though I couldn't recall it as soon as I awoke.

"Yeah, Armand, what's up?" What time is it, anyway? I'm trying to view the hour on my pager through the darkness.

"Hey, Steven. This guy came down to the ER with lower right quadrant pain, and it's a pretty good example of acute appendicitis. I've done the work-up on him but I think it would be good for you to come down and take a look at him."

"Sounds good, I'm on my way." It was ten past one. I had no idea where the ER was. Thank God there was a janitor when I hit the main lobby. He directed me there, and minutes later I was in front of Armand and our patient. Armand said that I didn't need to do a rectal exam, that had already been done, and that he just wanted me to see what an appendicitis looked like, I didn't need to page him when I was done, I could just head back upstairs.

I talked to the man, who had come in with his mother, and although he was obviously in a pretty fair amount of discomfort, he was keeping his spirits up and had a sense of humor about him. When he asked what an appendix was good for, I answered that it kept surgeons in business, and he laughed at that answer, but of course the laughing made him hurt. I didn't know if that was good bedside manner or a lousy time to play the comic.

I looked over Armand's notes as I was talking to the patient and his mother. They're both charming people, especially given the circumstances. I noted that he drank a heavy amount for someone in his late twenties and saw that Armand ordered liver function tests. One piece of history he gave stuck out at me, though. He said that he had had blood in his stools earlier in the day. I thought to myself, "Do you get bloody stools in appendicitis?" At that point I assumed that it was one little piece of information about appendicitis that I hadn't committed to memory. I finished up with them, told them that I was probably going to check up on him after his appendectomy, and wished them good night.

When I got back up to my room, I paged Armand. "Yeah, thanks for letting me come down, and I'm sorry if I just woke you up again, but I had a question," I said. "What's the deal with the bloody stools?"

"Funny you should say that, because I was thinking about that too," Armand replied. "I don't know what to make of that."

Well, that little light bulb in that medical brain of mine may be dim, but it functions allrighty. Still, I went to bed thinking that it was appendicitis. After all, Armand said it was. And I don't mean to be a smartass by saying that; he's three full years ahead of me in medical education, and he's seen a whole lot more cases than I have. Who was I to think it might be something else? By the morning, in between surgeries, I discovered that the CT scan didn't turn up any sign of appendicitis. It had to be something else, maybe a disease of the bowel known as "Crohn's disease," which a colonoscopy would confirm, or simply viral gastroenteritis. We missed the diagnosis, and I slept on it.

Thursday, July 13   pre-call

When I thought of surgery before my clerkship, I thought of the word *blood*. I imagined blood gushing everywhere, pumpers and sloshers shooting blood out of arteries, doctors scrambling furiously to prevent an OR geyser. I had been pretty disappointed, then, to see just how little blood is shed in a typical abdominal procedure (such as a gallbladder or appendix removal, or the repair of a hernia). I thought, "yeah, this is pretty cool, but when am I gonna see some really *messy* stuff going on?"

I got my wish yesterday morning. I had been scheduled to sit in on a laparascopic procedure that involved the kidney (although the general surgeons performing the surgery were careful not to use the word "kidney" on the OR schedule sheet, fearing that the urology docs would consider this poaching on their turf, since urologists specialize in doing surgery with the urinary tract system), but during pre-op the patient's EKG went loopy, so the surgery had to be cancelled for the day. I was somewhat bummed, and I went to my chief resident, and asked him what I should do. "Well, Dr. Fitzger is doing a thrombectomy over in 22," he said. "I suppose that's the best to make of a bad situation."

A thrombectomy. I'm going to have to hang around and see Fitzger pull a clot out of some guy's arm. *And* I haven't reviewed arm anatomy in a very long time. I thought: Oh, what a yawn.

Thankfully, I had one of the best experiences in surgery so far. Blood was going *everywhere* as we got into his axillary (upper arm) vein fishing around for the clot. That baby squirted, pumped, oozed, man was it great. Even better, Fitzger's resident was needed at another surgery, so I was left as his main assistant. Obviously I didn't do any sewing or cutting, it was Fitzger's show, but I got a great ringside seat and was responsible for keeping that vessel from pumping when he had to let go for whatever reason. The table was soaked in blood, my gown was half-covered in blood, Dr. Fitzger's hands were red with blood. I was having a blast.

The patient was a young man in end-stage renal disease. This had been his 40th time to have a clot removed. His entire upper left arm was almost one continuous scar from all of the cutting and suturing and re-cutting that had gone on. I think he knew from experiencing so many of these operations that the best defense against the horrible feeling before going under the knife was simply to have a sense of humor about the whole episode. He was flirting with the nurses, joking around with me, appearing to have a great time. Of course, he wasn't. At least some part of him had to be miserable, not only because he has had to endure that many invasions of his privacy by perfect strangers, but also that he wasn't likely to live to an old age.

I don't know enough about end-stage renal disease to tell you how long he is likely to live, but from my nascent education it looked like he could throw a clot from his legs up into his lungs any time, causing a possibly instantly-fatal embolism. And if an embolism won't kill him, something else surely will. Watching more elderly patients on the table, I don't feel as sorry for them or their families. I figure that even if they are in a terminal illness, they've had a lot of time to live and make meaning out of their lives. Their narratives have run most of their course anyway.

This guy, however, probably won't see his children and certainly not his grandchildren born. He's going to die before he can write an adequate story of his life. He's already had to endure an awesome amount of pain, I'm quite sure of that. What kind of hope can a doctor give to that patient? What really is our job in a case like that? Sure, we can come in and remove the clots, but sooner or later the disease is going to win out. What's our job then? I really have no idea.

$$\$\$\$\$\$\$\$\$\$$

Over at Team One it sounds like life is a much different beast. Today I was talking to a fellow student, Andathi, and we were swapping stories about what life in the OR for a med student is like. "Have you sat in on surgeries with the great Joshua Lipschitz?" I asked.

Joshua Lipschitz is a looming figure in the Cincinnati medical community. He is deeply respected and greatly feared. From the stories that I've heard, I've concluded that he is a megalomaniac. Lipschitz came here from one of the premiere institutions in the world and took a good surgery program and turned it into a great one, one of the top programs in the country. He has been the department chair for over twenty years, and is planning to step down once an appropriate replacement is found within the next year or two.

He is brilliant and driven, and expects the same out of all of his residents at all times — there is no time to take it easy while working on his watch. As a consequence, his program is filled with very smart, extremely hard-working, very uptight young physicians. And when he performs surgery, he considers it just that—a performance—and assumes that residents and students who have available free time will come and observe him in concert.

"Oh yeah, he's one of the main guys on the team," Andathi said. "We see him in surgery all the time. He does complicated stuff, some surgeries can last five, six, seven hours."

I thought *three* was an ungodly long time to stand. "So what's it like when he pimps you? Is it nerve-wracking?"

"Oh, we don't get pimped," Andathi said. "He never talks directly to med students."

"So you just sit there and watch?" I said.

"Pretty much. We're not allowed to speak unless we're spoken to."

Lipschitz appears to thrive on hazing his residents and interns. At the end of the intern year, all of the surgical interns take a national standardized exam. Lipschitz expects his interns to excel in this exam. My fourth-year resident Shelly, who is going to be a very good surgeon, did not apparently perform to his expectations. She had never spoken with Lipschitz outside of the operating room her entire intern year until those scores came back, when she was summoned to his office.

She entered the room, was told to sit down, and waited several minutes while he fiddled with some paperwork. Finally, he crossed his legs, folded his hands in his lap, looked directly at her, and said, "You know, you're stupid."

$$$$$$$$$

I could never be a surgeon for a multitude of reasons—the work is mostly technical rather than cerebral, the time spent standing is truly backbreaking, and many of the personalities are not as sunny as I prefer. That said, there is *one* part of nearly every surgery I love. When surgeons stitch, it is like watching a ballet. These people have stitched for so long that their movements are fluid, sparing, and deft. When there are *two* of them stitching simultaneously, as happened recently when I sat in on a thyroid surgery, I almost wanted to demand that someone play Mozart to complement the grace with which they were working.

Saturday, July 15   post-call

I had always thought of diabetes as a fairly benign disease, kind of like post-nasal drip — a nuisance to be sure, but not a devastating illness. During my second year I learned about the pathology of diabetes, but it never made a deep impression on me. It was just another disease to learn in a continuing parade of information to memorize.

Last night we admitted a patient for a severe toe infection. The man, a factory worker in his mid-forties, had been diagnosed with diabetes three months earlier when he noticed an infection on the sole of his foot after he had been walking about barefoot on a Lake Erie beach. The surgeon had to clean the wound by cutting off about half the skin on the sole of his foot because the infection was that widespread. Then three days ago, on the same foot, he stubbed his fourth toe and watched it get infected. He developed a fever and chills the next day, and had come in to see the surgeon again, who sent him directly to the Christ for admission.

When I saw the foot I was not entirely surprised to see a gangrenous toe with a dime-sized opening where the sterile packing had been placed between the fourth and fifth toe. The foot and calf were a bit red and definitely swollen, but I easily felt the pulses both on top of his foot and behind his ankle, which told me that the blood supply to the foot and toes was good. It didn't look very good, but I thought at the time that I had seen worse before med school during the regular course of my life. It wasn't pleasant to look at it but I wasn't going to wretch.

The next morning, Scott and Shelly joined Ross (the surgical intern) and me to take a look at the foot. Just as we were unwrapping the dressing, Dr. Basset, the attending surgeon who had admitted him, came in. We unwrapped the outer dressing, took off the gauze strips on the ulcer, and removed the packing. Shelly took a swab of the wound and (with gloves, of course) felt in between the fourth and fifth toe. I was astonished to see half her hand completely disappear up inside his foot. The man, who had no desire to watch the cleaning of the wound, was oblivious as he read the morning newspaper, keeping his eyes well protected from what was happening at the other end of the bed. A little bit of black tissue came out when her finger emerged as did bright red blood. Clearly this was a much larger wound than I had thought the night before. Now I knew why the surgeons were seeing him. We were evaluating him for amputation.

After we cut away the newly dead tissue, we cleaned the wound. It's hard to describe the sight of a wound that severe, with the tendon and bone of the toe easily visible once Shelly had cleared away the mess. But it's nearly impossible to describe the *smell* of it. At least for the foreseeable future, I will immediately associate the word "diabetes" with that smell. It's the smell I always associated with hospitals, and now after two weeks I was finally smelling it. I very nearly gagged.

At this point the question wasn't whether or not to save the foot, but just how best to prepare him to hear the news, which they were probably going to deliver in the next two or three days. The idea being that you don't just march back into his room and tell him what you know to be true, but you admit him for the weekend, and each time you see him on rounds you indicate that the toe's not doing well, and then the foot's not doing well, and then it's a grave situation. By that point he'll already started to have entertained the idea himself, and he's more prepared emotionally and intellectually to deal with what is clearly horrible news to someone who didn't have any apparent health problems only four months ago.

And this is only the *beginning* of his encounter with the medical system over the management of his disease. Unless he gets those blood sugars under serious control, things are going to get much, much worse. It's not that I didn't understand what I was reading about diabetes a few months ago. It's that I understand it in a much more visceral way now. There is a phrase I've been hearing from doctors all the time since I started medical school two years ago: *Once you see it, you never forget.* Now I see why.

$$$$$$$$$

Small things differentiate the classes of doctors. You'd think a doctor is a doctor, but within the profession each group often regards the other groups as different animals entirely. I'm in the elevator with Ross, I'm wearing my scrubs with my white coat, and we're in-between patients so I've got my stethoscope wrapped around my neck, where it's much more easily accessible. "Steven," Ross says, and then gestures to me to put my stethoscope in my front jacket pocket where I had seen all surgery residents put theirs.

"Sure. But why is it that you guys don't wear your stethoscopes around your neck?" I asked.

"Because that's what *medicine* docs do," he said with a clip of contempt.

Monday, July 17   8:00 p.m.

What, exactly, do I *do* in surgery?

The simplest answer is "I stand." Let's say the procedure is a partial gastric resection, where we cut part of the stomach out because of a lymphoma. Hopefully, I got around to reading a little bit about gastric lymphoma and stomach anatomy the night before. This is key because the *real* thing that I'm supposed to do during surgery is answer questions when they are directed at me. Questions aren't always directed at me, and half the time I spend just watching the proceedings, unless I ask questions of the attending, and given my legendary inability to keep my mouth shut, that often happens.

Back to the patient with gastric lymphoma. By the time we (the resident and I) arrive the patient is lying on the table, awake and usually very cold. I come over, hold the patient's hand as I introduce myself, and offer to get a warm blanket. Several minutes later the attending is present and this is when I'm in my most active role: Helping "prep" the patient for surgery.

This consists of strapping the patient's legs to the table so that they don't fall off during the procedure, shaving the belly so that there is no contamination by errant hairs, stuff like that. I try to put as much vim and vigor into the task as one can when one is placing tape on someone's abdomen, picking up all the loose hairs that have just been shaved off.

After scrubbing in at the sink and getting "gowned and gloved" by the OR techs, I move into third-year-student mode, meaning that I keep my mouth shut and wait to retract something. Next to standing, the only thing I do in vast quantity during a surgery is retracting. This means that I hold funny, spatula-shaped objects keeping various pieces of anatomy out of the way so that the surgeons can maintain a clear view of whatever it is that they're cutting and sewing. This part usually takes a few hours.

The time that I'm actually called upon to do something with a surgical instrument (other than hold it) is at the end, when we close the patient up. Typically the attending will ask the resident if they've got things under control, and they'll scoot out to dictate the procedure or go up to watch ESPN in the doctor's lounge. At that point, with the patient sewn up except for the layer of fat right beneath the skin, the kindly resident hands me the needle driver and I go to work. This lasts approximately three minutes, and we either sew up the skin layer with a subcutaneous stitch, which is very difficult for me to do, or we staple them, which is much easier. Surgery over, I follow the patient, anesthetist and the resident to the PACU, or "post-anesthesia care unit," and after about ten minutes there to make sure the patient is recovering without problems, I head for the lounge and wait for the next surgery.

Wednesday, July 19   5:30 p.m.   post-call

Last night, while I was on call, we did two emergency appendectomies within the span of about two hours. They were both white females in their early twenties and more-or-less had the classic signs of appendicitis. One of the women turned out to have a very sick abdomen, and when Shelly had opened her up she was looking around and concluded that the small intestine was so thick it could almost be confused with colon. The attending, Dr. Murphy, realized that the appendix probably wasn't the major offender. Instead, it was again Crohn's disease that was regarded as the likely culprit.

Appendectomies are emergency operations, but as emergencies go they're about as routine as surgeries get. So this young woman came into the hospital with her parents, suspecting that she had a condition that required a quick operation and would be home by the next day. Instead, she woke up to discover that she has a chronic, lifelong disease that may become much, much worse.

If the Crohn's gets bad enough, the small bowel can become obstructed. Once that happens, you have to go in and surgically remove the diseased portion. Each time you do that, you make it harder for the body to absorb all the nutrients coursing through the gut, since there's less gut to do the job. Worse yet, each resection increases the chance that another obstruction will occur. "The last thing you want to do with these patients is manage them surgically," Shelly said to me at about one-thirty last night, when we had finished the appendectomies. "Each time you go in, you up the chance that it will happen again, and it becomes a downward spiral. Eventually you've resected almost the whole small bowel and these people will end up having diarrhea every day for the rest of their lives." Or they'll have to take something called "TPN," which is a way of providing food directly into the blood without going through the digestive system, and creates its own host of problems. It works more-or-less, but it's not pleasant.

That's a worst-case scenario, and indeed many patients never have their Crohn's advance to that point. Yet this woman is potentially facing a life like I've described. All I kept thinking last night was: Her parents are out there in the waiting room thinking that their daughter is having a routine operation, obviously worried, but oblivious to the very heavy news that they're going to be hit with. I meant to ask Dr. Murphy how he broke news like that to the family, but I didn't find him today. I mean, Crohn's is a tricky piece of news to break. It's not like she has *cancer* and is in mortal danger, but it's not like she has the flu, either. How do you strike the balance between gravity and optimism?

Sunday, July 23

The board scores came back this week for the first 140 of us who took the Step One exam before June 18. A ridiculously high *nine* of us failed the exam. And we haven't even gotten back the final 20 scores.

I know a few of the people who failed. One of them is a young woman who, I have been told, had only used a slim book called *First Aid for the Boards* as a study guide. That seemed like a gargantuan mistake to me, and now I'm certain of it. In the front section, the authors of *First Aid* underscore that their book is *not* meant to be the sole source of review for a student. Their review material, which has maybe 15 pages of notes on each major section, is intended more to jog a student's memory as they consult *other* review sources. I personally used something on the order of 25 books and thousands of pages of notes.

For those nine people, they do not face a pleasant immediate future. First, they were removed from their clinical clerkships immediately. In order to finish med school on time, they have to retake the boards in late August, at which point they can return to their clinical rotations. The scores will be reported about four weeks later, and if they pass, they continue on, making up this summer rotation in the schedule-flexible fourth year. If they fail, they either have one chance to retake and start third year over again the following July, or they are finished with med school entirely, after two years of sweat and up to $60,000 in loans.

You have to understand that this test is a biggie among the hundreds of tests that medical students take to get where they want to go. It also illustrates the lengths to which numbers dictate the lives of medical professionals.

For instance, in order to just have a *chance* at getting into an average medical school in the United States, and University of Cincinnati basically fits that description, you first have to succeed in four basic science courses in college: Chemistry, biology, physics, and organic chemistry. You need to get, at absolute minimum, a 3.0 average in all of those courses, and to be truly competitive you really need at least a 3.4. Mind you, that's just to be competitive. A 3.0 probably won't get you into medical school, unless you are applying to a lesser-tier school or you smoke the MCAT — the Medical College Aptitude Test.

You also have to have a similar average in all your other classes as well, but a greater level of scrutiny is given to your science courses, and the higher your science GPA, the better chance you stand of getting in. Finally, if you're a "traditional" student (meaning that you go straight from college to med school), you take the MCAT, in the late spring of your junior year. MCATs cover those big four science courses, as well as a section on English. About 50,000 people take this test, and the national average is about a 24 (of a possible 45). If you want to get into med school, though, you better have a minimum of 27, and if you want to have a chance at getting into something above a lower-tier school, think 30 instead.

You may think: Well, there's some of the reason why doctors are such impersonal screwballs! All it takes to get into medical school is a numbers game! Where's the *humanity* in an admissions system like that?

The answer is that med schools do the best they can given that they can get up to 7,000 applications for every 150 positions available each year. They take the numbers and sift through those that they think have the potential to be good students. They may initially exclude a few thousand applicants, sending out a "secondary application" to those left, asking applicants to write an essay about how they want to save the world and stamp out disease. From these applications they get down to a working list of, say, six or seven hundred applicants, whom they invite to the school to interview.

Once you've gotten to the interview, you get scrutinized a good deal more carefully. (This is where jerks with 4.0s can come in too cocky and get booted — but I think that's a very rare occurrence.) In theory, this is where your "humanism" is appraised. In reality, even most psychopaths and boobs can manage to look normal for a few hours, judging from some of my classmates. From this group about three hundred offers are issued, and from that about 150 will accept (the others will usually accept an offer at another school).

The MCAT is probably a more important test than Step One in the grand scheme of things, since once you're into an American medical school you'll almost certainly find a residency and work somewhere, but Step One also dictates your future choices. You need, roughly speaking, a 179 to pass the exam. A 180, though, isn't necessarily cause for jubilation. You'll probably get a residency, but it could be in central South Dakota in Family Practice. Not that there's anything wrong with Family Practice or with living in South Dakota, but there might be something wrong with it if you were looking forward to a Dermatology residency in New York City.

You move up towards 200 and then you're into safer waters, and your choices expand somewhat. Many residency programs in pediatrics, internal medicine, and family medicine basically only care that you performed adequately, so unless you want to get into one of the most prestigious programs in these specialties, you can feel confident that you'll do well. Pass the 213-217 mark and you've beaten the mean, which may help you acquire a spot in some of the more competitive specialties such as emergency medicine or general surgery. Crank it up to 240 (about the top 6 or 7 percent) and you're starting to *dictate* your choices, provided that you're not a creep. The toughest residencies become attainable: Dermatology, radiology, ophthalmology, orthopedics — specialties with big-time incomes and pretty easy hours. Get a 271, like one classmate of mine, and you've gotten a score in the top one percent, and if you have any social skills whatsoever, you probably don't even need to apply to more than a few programs in even the most competitive fields where highly qualified applicants routinely submit upwards of 30 applications.

For what it's worth, before I got to med school I was at best a marginal candidate. I had a 3.1 science GPA, but did pretty well on my MCATs with a 31. That's not a very good risk to take if you're a med school, though my age, unusual background as an

English teacher, and some very good recommendations helped me. But I applied to 21 medical schools, got four interviews, and was only admitted here.

Since I've come to med school my numbers have evened out and I'm doing about what an average med student should do. Obviously I was not among those nine fails. I had set out to beat the national mean, and that's exactly what I did: I got a 219. With those numbers I won't get into a residency at Mass General Hospital or at Johns Hopkins[*], but I have a pretty good sense of what kind of a med student I am, which is to say I'm an average one, at least as far as the scientific and medical knowledge part of it goes. Whether or not I have the social intangibles that will help me excel remains to be seen.

Tuesday, July 25 pre-call

After a ventral hernia repair this morning I headed up to the surgery library to do some studying, figuring that I'd be off until everyone gets back together at two or three to do afternoon rounds. I got paged by Ross at about one-thirty. "Hey, come down to twenty-one," was all his message said.

I got down posthaste and it was a surgeon that I had never worked with, a brand-new attending named Hasbro who had just finished the University residency. It was yet another lap cholecystectomy, at this point probably my twentieth. We got all set up, put the camera in just beneath the man's navel, and what I saw on the monitor I had never seen before. All the other gallbladders that I've looked at looked basically the same, but this one was swollen (the others looked like a balloon that had deflated slightly) and white (the others were a dark-green). This was one sick-looking gallbladder. Was an attending only weeks out of finishing residency going to be able to handle this thing?

As it turned out, the answer would be "no." They stuck a needle in to extract some of the contents of the gallbladder so that they could grasp it better with their laparoscopic instruments, but that only went so far. I couldn't even tell

---

[*] This turned out to be a very accurate prediction. You can see how I fared at competitive programs in my chosen field in the epilogue.

the *area* where the cystic duct was, and usually I can see the duct itself. It was hard to tell where the gallbladder ended and the colon wall began. My job in this, as was my job in all lap procedures, was to hold the camera. Soon it became clear that additional expert help would be needed, and I heard Hasbro ask for somebody but I missed the conversation, focused as I was on doing my camera job. Two minutes later, a tall man poked his head in the door, and said, "Hey, Scott, I hear there's some problems with this gallbladder."

EVIL DOCTOR BLASTON!

There I am, *actively* trying to avoid working with this man on my final week at Christ so that I can avoid being yelled at, and he *still* manages to come in on a case. Blaston's dropping in to say hello quickly turned into Blaston's scrubbing in, and before I know it, I'm camera-driving on *his* operation. "Come in, *come in*," he's saying to me, and I think, it's nice to know he's consistent. Then, a new line. "Listen, would you *please* keep the camera above the fat so that I can see?"

You bet, big man.

It's just part of my personality to get defensive when I hear a tone like his. I know that I shouldn't take it personally but inevitably a part of me feels like a dog that's just been kicked in the gut. When I came up to the lounge afterwards I spoke with my classmate Jason, who had done Blaston's regularly scheduled surgeries today. How was it, I asked.

"Today? Oh, today was a good day," Jason said. "I only got yelled at *once*. He said, 'Can't you keep the damn camera in the center of the field so I can see what I'm doing?' I felt pretty good since that's all he said."

Jason, you've got a lap nephrectomy with Blaston tomorrow, and I'm doing a lap cholecystectomy with Basset. It was your choice. More power to you.

Saturday, July 29

Yesterday I finished my month of surgery at Christ. I have the weekend off and then I start at the VA on Monday for a month there.

Instead of finishing on a high note, I was seriously humbled — a feeling I've become accustomed to by now. This past Wednesday morning I had scrubbed in on a case with him for about the twentieth lap chole of the month. I liked lap choles in that I was playing an active role by holding the camera, but I didn't like them in that I wasn't learning anything after the third time I did it. But that morning Dr. Basset decided to do, one full month and twenty lap choles into my rotation, what no other surgeon had thought to do. He decided to ask me questions about cholecystitis, or gallbladder inflammation. I *thought* I was on safe ground on this topic, having reviewed it on a few occasions preparing for these surgeries, but I learned pretty quickly that I had learned *facts* but hadn't made the necessary *connections* between them to be of any use to me.

So you think it through: A woman comes into your office, complaining of "right upper quadrant," pain (that's pain above and to the right of the navel: We divide the gut into four basic regions based on their relation to it). It's a vague but intense kind of pain, not sharp in character. She's forty-three, and she tells you that she's often felt this pain after she eats food, especially fatty food. Three nights ago she had fried chicken and mashed potatoes, and the pain started but this time it didn't quit. What, doctor, do you do? This was a no-brainer to me: The major cause of cholecystitis is gallstones, and the way to diagnose gallstones is by performing an ultrasound. So that's what I said: Do an ultrasound.

Basset halted. "Don't you want to do a history and physical before doing an ultrasound?" he asked. Yeah, sure. "Well, what would you want to know from her history?" Hmmm. I had to pause to think. You see, I had thought like this: *Cholecystitis → ultrasound → lap chole.* But that's the easy part of the thought process. I wasn't thinking through the tough part, which is how do you *get* to the diagnosis. The woman didn't come in with cholecystitis, she came in with RUQ pain. How can I be so sure that it wasn't something else? What else could it be? *That's* why you take a history and physical, because (so my superiors tell me constantly) 90 percent of the time a good, thorough history will give you a diagnosis or a short list of the two or three most likely candidates.

Back to my problem. "You'd want to know if she has any history of recent travel," I say, thinking of hepatitis or other, stranger infectious diseases that affect the liver, diseases which are almost always acquired when people travel to "exotic" places. Basset informs me that this woman is classic Cincinnati—meaning that she has never left home in her life. Hmmm. Seconds are elapsing. Basset suggests that maybe I'd like to ask something about her *stools*. A-Ha! The stools! I readily agree. Yes, tell me about the stools. Well, what do you want to *know* about the stools, Basset asks me. Hmmm. I think for the obvious: Any blood? Nope, no blood. Hmmm. I realize that I have no earthly idea what he's driving at.

He was driving at this: The reason why your excrement is brown is because of the gallbladder's product, bile. Bile itself is a golden-yellow liquid, but it empties into the intestines, and bacteria living in your gut digest it, and as the nutrients & liquids of food are slowly taken away, what's left is a brown, semi-solid mass. Block that bile duct, though, and your stools won't have that brown color anymore, they'll turn a bluish-gray ("clay-colored," the medical texts say, which caused me a great deal of confusion, because when I think of clay I see a terra-cotta rusty red). This woman's stools *did* change colors, but didn't think of it until you mentioned it to her. Still that bile's gotta go somewhere if it didn't get into the intestines, so where'd it go? I realize, with painful slowness, that it has to go into the *veins*, and from there to the *arteries*, where there's going to be higher blood levels which the kidneys will try to filter out, so there's going to be that bile-brown color to her *urine*.

That paragraph took you maybe thirty seconds to read, it took me five minutes to figure out, and I had to have Basset and Ross lead me by the nose to understand. Then the *real* fun began. "What, besides *exotic* liver disease," he asked, "should you be thinking about in your differential?" By this stage, I was feeling so turned around in my head that even answers I knew weren't coming to me, and Dr. Basset's impatience grew with each passing question I did not answer correctly.

His tone remained even throughout, but he said to me, "Steven, do they still teach pathology at the med school?" and, "Steven, I really think you need to do some reading," and, "Steven, you need to start thinking like a clinician." I was feeling pretty small after that surgery. But I did learn a valuable lesson that I think will help me in the coming months. You have to see things from the point of view of the patient coming into your office (or the ER, or the wards, etc.) to think about what diseases they could have in order to make the proper diagnosis. Because if you don't, you won't know what questions to ask, and if you don't ask the right questions, you might not get an important clue which will guide you toward that diagnosis. They said this last year, but now I get it: Patients will not simply volunteer up information, you have to ask it to get it out of them.

All that happened Wednesday morning. I was on call on Wednesday night, and I thought I'd have a great chance to do some studying and get some sleep. After all, the last two times I was on call I was busy doing emergency appendectomies and exploratory surgeries for small bowel obstructions. What were the odds that I was going to be in midnight surgery again? I went from the OR in the morning to class in the afternoon, and then I came back to Christ at 5:30 and paged Ross. He was down in OR 15, and said I had better high tail it down there.

Dr. Caffey was in a surgery that had begun at noon and was scheduled to be over at four. It was nearly six when I walked in and it became clear that Caffey was in a foul mood, because six hours into the surgery they hadn't even found the root of the problem. I wasn't of much help, but one doesn't just walk out of the OR when an attending surgeon is at work, especially Caffey, who is a Team One doctor over at the U. So I stood there over Caffey and Shelly while Caffey cursed at Shelly every time she used the electric scalpel. Caffey would hold her fingers underneath the tissue that she wanted cut, and Shelly would dutifully turn the scalpel on, it would burn through the tissue, and go right down onto Caffey's fingers, shocking her, which would cause a half-minute out burst: *Fuck! Jesus Christ, Shelly! Why the fuck can't you operate a Bovie? You're a fourth year*

44

resident, for crying out loud! You're killing me! I'm serious, Shelly, you're killing me!

Then she'd calm down again, they'd do some more holding, poking, probing, and then I'd hear Caffey say, "Bovie," and I stepped back, not wanting to look, aware of the impending catastrophe. BLAM! Caffey's screaming at Shelly again. This went on for something like two, three hours. I said practically nothing, did practically nothing except watch Caffey scream at everyone in sight, and we finally finished up about 10:30 with a very sick woman getting wheeled off to recovery.

Shelly and I retired upstairs to the OR lounge where we found Ross, who was ready to tell me that we had an emergency lap appendectomy with…? Yes, you guessed it, the same Dr. Basset that I had managed to impress so much earlier in the day.

Basset told me that this surgery was really a two-person job, so I could just watch the surgery on the TV monitor, and he'd "make sure to ask some questions." I thought, "Oh God, here it comes again." Nice circularity on the day, though — start out the day feeling incompetent, end the day feeling incompetent. I was feeling like a million bucks.

Once the camera got into the abdomen, Basset asked me to describe it. I said it was swollen and inflamed. He then wanted to know what word I would use to describe the material on the outer rim of the appendix. It was white. I assumed he was asking about the anatomy of the appendix, so I told him it was the serosa. "The serosa?" he quipped, "I don't think so." I wasn't sure what he was driving at, so I suggested that it was the omentum. "Omentum?" He swung the camera toward the yellow omentum and asked, "Now does *this* look the same color as that appendix?" No, it didn't. I apologized and said I wasn't sure what he was asking.

"Are you familiar with the term 'exudate'?"

Exudate is the term that describes purulent, pus-like discharge. It is white and filled with the remnants of dead white blood cells, and other organic debris. It's the stuff you see in zits. Then Basset popped a forty-megaton zit on *me*.

"Steven, I'm *really* not sure that you took pathology." He then became silent, and proceeded to ignore me for the next hour and a half. During this time, I built my rage up to exquisite heights. I imagined doing some surgery on *him*, the miserable bastard. Of course it was exudate. That wasn't a fair question. If he had said, "What's the term used to describe the discharge from the appendix?" I'd have gotten it instantly, but he asked the question in such a vague way I had to guess what it was that he was looking for. Now I was being *punished*, completely left in silence to ponder my *stupidity*, all caused by a bungled question not of my own making. I was furious, and impotent to do anything about it. As he tried to drop the appendix into this specialized plastic mini-bucket, he was having a great deal of difficulty, and I felt like God was granting me a little indirect gotcha-back. Thank you, Jesus.

Just when I'm convinced that they're going to finish up and he's going to walk out of the room without so much as another word to me, he says, "Steven — what would you want me to do if we had seen a normal looking appendix?"

"You'd still take it out." Why? he asked. "Because once you're inside, you still want to remove the appendix, since it serves no important physiological function and you don't want to have to go in again to remove it at a later date."

Would you want to do anything else?

"Sure, you'd want move the camera around to see if there was any evidence of a different disorder that might have caused the pain that mimicked appendicitis. You'd first want to see if there was any evidence of Crohn's disease, so you'd look at the small bowel for thickening and swelling. If it's a female you're operating on, which in this case applies, you'd want to look at the internal female genitalia to see if there is any evidence of ectopic pregnancy, although at forty-five she's a little old for that, or pelvic inflammatory disease, or…um….polycystic ovaries. All of those disorders can first appear as right lower quadrant pain."

"*Now* you're thinking like a clinician!" came his swift response. Redemption.

Humiliation aside, it was the biggest leap in my clinical education thus far. I got my first glimpse at *how* to think like a doctor. Basset was tough on me but fair, and his reasoning was right. The point of medical school is not to memorize loads of information. Because we are given so much to memorize, that point is easy to forget. The real use of a medical education is to be able to *think clinically*, which means put those learned facts together in a way that serves a patient well. That day was the first day I really thought that way, and all credit was due to Dr. Basset. (Though, truth be told, I was still pleased to see that he had to struggle to get that appendix in the plastic basket.)

Saturday, August 5   VA Hospital

If hospitals were cars, Christ Hospital would be a Nissan — no-nonsense, nice handling, a good mid-level car. The Veteran's Administration Hospital would be a rusting 1976 Dodge Dart.

The vets put up with a level of discomfort that would be unheard of at one of the private hospitals. They'll sleep three men in a 10 x 20 foot room with virtually no privacy and only one television set. That may not sound so bad, but *you* try going to sleep when your roommate has the baseball game on at 11:00 p.m., and the nurses are coming in to draw blood on your other roommate, who happens to insist on keeping the door open, which shines the light directly in on *you*.

Despite these inconveniences, not to mention the fact that many of these men (and a few women) suffer from truly horrible diseases, most of the Vets are remarkably high-spirited, all things considered. You'll see guys who have had half their colon removed, they're throwing up once or twice a day, fainting when they get up to go to the commode, and "eating" *Ensure* chocolate-flavored nutrition shakes, and every time you come around to see them they'll light up, with big smiles on their faces, and say, "You're the best, doc! I got all the confidence in the world in you!"

It may be that these men, due to their service in the military, are used to such crowded conditions. It may also be that many of them are receiving health care that they otherwise might not have had they stayed at home and worked at low-paying menial jobs that never offered them a chance at adequate health insurance. And they may not know the difference, not ever having slept in a clean, spacious suburban hospital. No matter the cause, I like these guys, and I like the VA. It's a very warm environment despite the hassles, and it reminds me a great deal of the camp I worked at during my college years, which was very spartan, but you never much thought about the lack of creature comforts because you were too busy enjoying your work and the people you worked with.

VA Team One is led by the fifth-year chief Resident Brad Crafton, a tall, surly character with a strawberry-blond mustache. Aside from the mustache, Crafton is what I picture when I picture a surgeon. He never smiles, rarely encourages, and is ready with a sharp reply if you make one verbal misstep.

I'm on Team Two, which is led by Bart Gilliam, a chief from somewhere in the south, whose spine seems so thoroughly beaten down after five years of surgery that he looks like a walking question mark. Bart's good with the patients and good with us. Each morning that we've had time to eat breakfast after rounds he's done brief teaching sessions with us about various issues in surgery. But he, too, can be terse with us. We asked him when we could check to see what surgeries were being performed, and he said quickly, "Hey, you can read a schedule as easily as I can." Well, shucks, boss, that's true, but *where's* the schedule?

Working under these two Aryan-looking gentlemen is Parat Bindot, an intern of either middle-eastern or Indian heritage; Eric Rodriguez, a Texan with some Latino background; and Richard White, an African-American from Maryland. It's an all-American portrait.

$$$$$$$$$

By walking around the VA and poking your head in patient rooms, whether those patients are on the surgery service or not, you get a vivid glimpse of Ways You Don't Want To Die. To see one or two really sick patients at Christ is merely temporarily uncomfortable, because you're mostly surrounded by patients who are coming in for quick hernia repairs, gallbladders removals, thyroidectomies. In theory, most of the Christ patients will get better and return to a normal life. Not so the VA patients. Nearly *all* of the surgical cases have conditions that you don't ever, ever want to get.

Take the vascular cases, which make up a good chunk of the patients in the hospital right now. There are several patients who can't get any blood to their feet, and so even minor trauma that we regard as mere inconvenience, like stubbing one's toe, can lead to an infection that threatens the entire foot, or worse. My first patient was a gentleman who had lost blood supply to his toes, but never developed an infection. Thus, instead of the putrid, foul appearance of a typical infected, poorly-perfused foot, his toes simply mummified. On my second day on service we took him into the OR and basically sawed off the dead parts. It was not a finesse procedure. Now half the surface of the part of the foot that remains is a gaping open wound.

If this seems unpleasant it runs a distant second to another patient on the service, one with esophageal cancer. Esophageal cancer is to my thinking about one of the worst ways to exit this earth. Typically the first thing patients notice is having a difficult time swallowing, because the tumor has become so large it closes off the esophagus. By that point, the tumor is so advanced the chances of surviving it are pretty poor. Worse, as they die of the disease, they continue to have problems getting food, and they have nausea, vomiting, diarrhea — in effect their entire quality of life goes south.

These diseases have one thing in common: They have similar associated risk factors, mainly smoking and alcohol consumption. It's difficult to get esophageal cancer without smoking or drinking, and while you can have vascular problems without smoking or drinking, it doesn't make matters any better and almost certainly contributes to the severity of the disease. The overwhelming majority of VA patients on the surgery service either smoke or drink or do both, and do so in more-than-moderate quantities. If you ever have a child that has begun to smoke and you want to convince them that that's not a good decision, send them over to the VA to have a look at the guys with vascular trouble. And I haven't even mentioned the patients that have emphysema and lung cancer, who are largely confined to the internal medicine service.

Thursday, August 10

Despite a great deal of worrying I've done in the past week about my evaluation, I did just fine, at least at Christ. I got my written evaluation on Tuesday, and my marks put me at the border of Honors. This means that if I do well on my oral and written exams, I could get Honors, but if I really screw up then I get only a pass. Plus I still get my VA evaluation.

The evaluations were something of a mystery to me. My evaluation from Silverman was basically what I expected—my "fund of medical knowledge" was impressive to him, and while I don't think that's true in reality I knew I impressed him because I fortunately had the time to prepare well for his cases. But he only gave me average marks for my rapport with patients and staff, which I thought was not only above average but also plain to see.

Even more strange, though, was that my second evaluation was written by a Dr. Bellamy, a surgeon in semi-retirement. I haven't written anything about Bellamy because I have had only cursory interactions with him; we literally only met once and shook hands. For a man who had never met me, he had a paragraph's worth to say, and I fell just one point shy of getting an Honors. Guess I must have made one hell of an impression.

I figure there's three explanations for how a medical student could get an evaluation from a total stranger who never got to see the student in action. One possibility is that he asked those who had worked with me—the residents, the chief, other attendings—and then extracted the general feel of the comments and judged from there. Another possibility is that the attending physicians deliberately give you a grade that puts you on a borderline for High Pass or Honors; thus it's the responsibility of the *student* to make or break their grade based on their written and oral exam performance.

The third possibility is that there's no rhyme or reason to the system at all and those attendings who can't properly evaluate a student just Make Stuff Up.

Wednesday, August 16

Last night was my call night, and what a night it was. I got introduced to what it's like to work with patients with HIV, and it scared the shit out of me—a reaction that I would scarcely have believed I would feel. You see, I like to think I am fairly well read on HIV. I have met HIV positive people. I am not burdened by the fears of HIV that complicated relationships between doctors, nurses, and patients in the early years of the epidemic. But I have never sutured a profusely bleeding scalp wound on an HIV positive man, which is precisely what happened yesterday evening.

We were called down to the ER for two surgery consults, the first a patient with a scalp laceration. He was an African-American man in his thirties with HIV, was intoxicated and had apparently been beaten by an acquaintance. We had learned as first-year students in gross anatomy that scalp lacerations bled profusely because the scalp was held taut by very tough connective tissue. While it *looked* bad, we were assured, it was only a superficial wound and that, unless there was a cranial fracture, it was a relatively simple problem to fix. When I saw this gentleman's head I knew why we had been given the advice not to freak out. There was bright red blood oozing out of a cut about half an inch long, and I wondered for the life of me how I was going to place a suture in that wound with nowhere to put the stitch except his skull.

I found out that answer pretty quickly: I was going to *staple* the cut after I cleaned the wound and gave him some injections of local anesthetic. That was the first time I had ever given an injection of local. When you see someone else do it, it looks pretty simple—point and shoot. It turns out to be more difficult, although perhaps that was because I had to work with the scalp, which didn't yield well, and after I put the needle in and depressed the plunger I felt strong resistance.

The only way that I knew that any local was going in was because I could see the fluid displacing his own poisonous blood, which was streaming off his head and onto the gauze pads, the bed, the sheets, you name it.

It didn't help that this was my first real case of closing a wound. I had closed several wounds in the OR, but that's a relatively low-pressure affair, when the patient is asleep, won't move, and can't feel the pain. You can mess up, drive a stitch right through the patient's skin, realize that you've gone too deep or too shallow, and start over again. Messing up when the patient is awake is a good deal more frightening, even if they are under a local anesthetic. In addition, this gentleman was drunk, clearly upset that a man he considered his friend had badly hurt him, and was staring up at two white doctors holding needles. There was no way to know if he was going to decide at any moment that it was time to get up and bolt, and if he was going to do that when my eyes or mouth were exposed.

However, aside from the moments when we were injecting him with the local, when he merely voiced his discomfort, he hardly moved or made a peep. I placed four staples, cleaned up his wound, tried to comfort him as best I could, and hastily made a retreat. Although I couldn't understand much of what he said, it was clear that he very much appreciated the work that we did for him. "You docs are great," he stammered, and I felt pretty crappy since I was so uncomfortable with the situation and so scared of him.

The second patient, Mr. Aikenhead, who had a bypass graft placed in his right leg three weeks before, had returned complaining of a severe pain in his thigh where the incision was. When you examine a patient like that, under some circumstances, you don't put gloves on. Eric started to take a look at the leg without gloving, and Brad said, "Eric, I think you should put some gloves on." Eric looked up and immediately understood what Brad meant. At first I assumed that he was just being the chief, correcting his residents on basic universal precautions. Only after the resident covering the ER explained that the patient was HIV-positive did I understand the import of Brad's command.

It turned out that just lightly touching Mr. Aikenhead on the leg could cause him to scream. Brad got a needle and an 18-gauge syringe and proceeded to stick the needle directly into his thigh around the wound. *That* got a response. Mr. Aikenhead hollered. He slowly filled the 50cc syringe filled with a red, clearish-looking fluid. He withdrew the needle and syringe, handed it to Eric, and repeated the process with a new needle and syringe. This time bright red blood emerged into the syringe, and Brad detached the needle from the syringe, keeping the needle inserted into the thigh so that he could just screw in another syringe. He repeated this five or six more times. By the end of it, Mr. Aikenhead was sitting up, almost smiling, and talking directly to Brad and Eric, thanking them for taking away the pain. It was a complete—and from my perspective a wholly unanticipated—transformation.

The drainage helped him temporarily, but the obvious problem became what to do with his leg, since he clearly had a bleeder in there somewhere. Brad called Giancolo, the attending, to see whether or not we should simply open him up immediately. Giancolo said to follow him for the next hour and see what happens, maybe we could sit on it for the night and we won't have to do anything. An hour later, Mr. Aikenhead was screaming again, and even I could see that his leg had swollen up.

Same routine with the needle and syringe, with the same outcome. We had to repeat this process yet again before we finally wheeled him into the OR. We finally got to the OR at about 1:30 a.m. when Giancolo and the anesthetist had arrived. As we were preparing him for the surgery, Giancolo pulled on the bandage that had been covering the incision, and suddenly *SPLOOSH!* A stream of blood shot five feet across the room. I came over to put pressure on it while Giancolo, Brad, and Eric scrubbed in. I had never been so scared by just holding my index finger on something, like it was a bomb.

Once they opened him up, it was a pretty simple operation. They found the bleeders, sewed them up, extensively flushed the area, removing all the clots that had accumulated, and closed him again. Giancolo even found time to pimp me, of all things, at 2:30 in the morning, the first time he'd ever spoken to me. "What do you do when someone comes in bleeding?" he asked.

"Find the bleeder," I said immediately. Seemed logical.

"No."

Silence. Then I realize I do know the answer. "Oh—you want to stabilize the patient. Give him two large-bore IVs and give him one or two liters of lactated Ringer's."

"Or saline. Then what?"

"Ummm...find the bleeder?"

Irritation on surgeon's face in the middle of the night. "Well, *what* did you do when we were prepping him?"

I realize that I know *this* answer, too. "Put direct pressure on the site to prevent further bleeding while you prep him."

"Mmmmm," growled Giancolo in the affirmative.

And so it went. We finished at about four, when I was finally able to go to the bathroom for the first time in six hours, and went to bed to get two and a half hours of sleep before morning rounds.

Thursday, August 17

Dr. Manning gave a lecture to us on Thursday about abdominal wall hernias. He's a tough guy—good-looking in a macho sort of way, with very short-cropped hair and a posture that communicates utter confidence. He's also an Air-Force alumnus and a Trauma Surgeon, which is the ultimate macho field in surgery.

"What are the six rules of surgery?" he asks.

"Don't mess with the pancreas," says Josh, an MD/PhD student.

"That's number four," Manning replies. The pancreas, the geographic center of the human body, is the crossroads of all sorts of anatomy: Liver, spleen, stomach, intestines, aorta. Poking around in that area is unwise unless it's absolutely necessary. Plus Mr. Pancreas doesn't like to be jostled about by a surgeon's hands, and he often causes tremendous postoperative pain for his owner if this takes place.

Nobody can offer any other suggestions. "Okay, guys, here they are. Rule number one: If you can eat, eat. Rule number two: If you can sleep, sleep. Rule number three: If there's pressure, then relieve it. Rule number four: Don't mess with the pancreas. Rule number five: Do *not* sit in this" — he points directly to the seat that Joshua Lipschitz sits in — "chair. Someone in the surgery clerkship always manages to do that in their first week. Rule number six: When you buy candy, make sure it is not divisible."

Meaning that everyone will pounce upon you and eat your hard-won M & Ms.

Sunday, August 20 5:00 p.m.

A surgical dictum: The only time you don't perform a rectal exam is when you do not have a finger, or the patient does not have an anus. Rectal exams are, obviously, the least liked part of the physical examination by medical students, residents, attendings, and most of all the patients. But at the VA, especially in the clinics, where we see a high volume of patients, medical students are *always* the ones required to perform the necessary task.

This is fine. Ever since I performed my first few rectal exams, I no longer feel embarrassed or squeamish. But what we're doing in there is still often a mystery. I don't have the slightest clue what a cancerous prostate feels like, or how to tell the difference between hardened stool in the upper rectum and a mass. It's a little scary to perform this exam, knowing that some of the less vigilant residents might simply take our word that so-and-so has a "normal" prostate, deferring to the word of someone who has felt maybe ten or fifteen prostates.

It reminds me of a story from my first year of medical school. At the end of the first year, UC students spend one afternoon a week for a few months working with a "real" doctor in a "real" doctor's office. My doc was a urologist, and after a week or two he started to walk me through rectal exams on patients who were willing to oblige. He'd quiz me about how this prostate felt, or how large that prostate seemed, and I felt as if I were being asked to read hieroglyphics. I had no idea how to answer. After one of these quizzes, I asked him about his learning curve. "Doctor, it all feels pretty much the same to me. How many prostates did you feel before you were really confident that you knew what was going on?" I asked.

"Oh, about a thousand or two," was his nonchalant reply.

Monday, August 21   post-call

Q: What's the difference between a third-year medical student and a bucket of shit?
A: The bucket.

Q: What's the difference between a third-year medical student and a pile of shit?
A: People try to avoid stepping on the pile.
—jokes from various residents

In the past two weeks, I've come to understand that VA patients will perform heroic feats of self-abuse to get their bodies into the kind of shape that require our intervention. The body, I am beginning to think, is a pretty resilient piece of machinery. You can bang it up, overstuff it with lousy food, dump various toxic chemicals into it via injection, drink, or smoke, and usually it will (in the manner of Timex) just keep on ticking. Most of the people who have shown up at the VA for help have gone one step too far.

Take "Scorpion," for instance. That's the preferred name of Mr. William Gaskill, a 49 year-old construction worker from Louisville with a very large tattoo of a scorpion on his right forearm alongside a tattoo of the Nazi "SS" and opposite a large left-arm tattoo of a swastika. There's another tattoo on his leg, but I can't make it out; it was "damaged" four months ago when he had coronary bypass surgery and took a vein out of his leg. He's missing well over half his teeth, and his thin black hair reaches his shoulders. Despite the Nazi skin decorations, he's actually a pleasant guy. "How do you feel this morning?" I ask Mr. Gaskill. "With my *fingers*!" is his immediate response.

Scorpion came to us for the removal and biopsy of a lung mass, which the doctors feared was cancer. In addition to his heart and lung trouble, he suffered from intermittent claudication, a condition that prevents one from walking far distances without great pain. That may also need surgical correction at a later date, but first we had to find out what the mass in his lung was. If it was small-cell cancer, fixing his legs wouldn't matter much, because the odds that he'd be dead in five years were pretty high.

I interviewed him right before the operation, and I wanted to know about his smoking history. In medicine, we have a concept of the total smoking burden called the "pack-year." If you smoked one pack a day for five years, you have a five pack-year history, or if you smoked two packs in the same time, then you have a ten pack-year history. The pack-year idea is based on the concept that the overall length of time and the amount of cigarettes smoked are of equal importance in determining one's risk for various lung diseases, but especially cancer. Last year, when I was learning how to take a patient's history, I had encountered a man with a sixty pack-year history, and I thought that was impressive. The week before I interviewed Scorpion, I had met two men in their late-seventies who had easily managed to outperform that: They had *one hundred fifty* pack-year histories!

Mr. Gaskill had managed to equal the pack-year histories of these gentlemen at age *forty-nine*. He had begun smoking at age six, and within a few years was up to several packs a day, topping off at six packs a day until he went in for his heart surgery. I don't know exactly how many cigarettes are in a pack, but I assume it's about 20. So that's 120 cigarettes a day, and an average waking day is about sixteen hours. My math says that's a smoke, on average, every eight minutes of every day of over forty years. That's impressive.

What's more impressive is that each of his three brothers — all with smoking histories comparable to Scorpion's — never made it past 50. His father managed to eke it out to 57. Their deaths did not appear to provide enough of an incentive to quit, and I'm not sure that the heart surgery did, either; one of the nurses warned me not to walk too far with him for fear that he'd drag me outside and borrow cigarettes off the nearest smoker, as there's always someone (often nurses) hanging around the entrance of the VA smoking cigarettes.

Tuesday, August 22

This is the last week of the clerkship, the payoff pitch as it were. Today began the most harrowing exercise of these past two months, namely the oral examinations. They're spread out over Tuesday, Wednesday, and Thursday — mine is tomorrow — and everyone's been in a panic for about the past week. I've spent virtually every night eating dinner with Andrea (one of my closest friends in the school and who happens to be doing her surgery clerkship as well) the two of us relentlessly grilling each other on possible questions that they might ask of us: What are the Duke's criteria for staging colon cancer? What are the presentations of Leriche's syndrome? Can you define the borders of Hesselbach's triangle? And on, and on, and on. This is a major reason why I haven't written a lick, and why, logically, I've chosen the night before the exam to scrawl some notes.

I think it's safe to say that the vast majority of the 24 students taking surgery right now are mildly terrified of the orals. To have a mediocre performance on a written exam is a relatively anonymous affair; to make a complete fool of yourself in front of your superiors, to actually *demonstrate* your frank ignorance of surgery in front of the most hard-core, intimidating doctors in the business, is enough to send one scurrying under a bed for several days. Hopefully I've used this to my advantage, in that profound fear of disgrace has served as an incentive.

Additionally, I had a powerful motivational experience last Thursday. One of the burn surgeons offered a brief "how to prepare for the orals" session. I figured that this was a nice, touchy-feely gesture, and anyone who donates his own valuable time must be one of the cuddliest surgeons around. When he entered the room, he gave some introductory remarks about topics that we were likely to be questioned on (study breast cancer a lot more than gastric carcinoma, for instance), how to maintain poise, etc. Then he asks for a volunteer to simulate the experience, and *gives* us the diagnosis in advance: "Oh, let's do something simple, like an appendicitis." I figured this was a good chance to hone my skills, and after all, I knew about appendicitis. So I volunteered to be the mock examinee. What could be the downside?

The downside, I would quickly discover, is that I would be totally humiliated in front of all of my classmates. I repeated, point-for-point, the mistakes I made with Dr. Basset over a month ago. *Woman, age 17, comes into the ER, and she's got abdominal pain, what do you do?* Where's the pain, I ask. *It's in her right lower quadrant.* Does she have rebound tenderness, I ask. *Yes, she does.* Let's take her to the OR, I offer, and my mind is trying to anticipate his questions about the anatomy of the appendix and colon.

"What?!" Dr. Burn Surgeon asks. "That's *all* you want to find out in her history? My goodness, young man, I don't want *you* anywhere near me with a knife!" My classmates are quietly chuckling and suddenly my mind is whirring. I stutter and stammer and try to think of questions to ask her in the history — travel history, last menstrual period, bloody stools — but I'm just throwing out whatever comes to mind, I'm no longer thinking in any organized manner. I'm sweating furiously. Each time I offer a question he says, "Okay, is that it?" Finally, as I run out of questions that I can think of, he starts humming the tune to *Jeopardy* during the silence. More chuckles, more sweat. Finally, I say that I'm done with questions, I think she's got appendicitis (clever!), let's get her to the OR.

He looks upward at the ceiling. "Lord, why do you do this to me?" he asks. "Do you mean to tell me that you don't want to perform a *physical exam* on her, and you don't feel it necessary to draw any *labs* or get any *studies*?" Everyone's laughing now, me included — me only because I didn't know what else to do, like I farted loudly in the middle of a Joshua Lipschitz lecture.

And on it went, for another five minutes. I spent the rest of the review session not paying attention to the other questions, instead mulling over my stupidity, and the casual arrogance that led me to be the first volunteer, idiotically thinking I'd knock it out of the park on what was, after all, a simple trial run, with the diagnosis *given* to me in advance. I did nothing over the weekend except make long flowcharts for almost every major surgical situation that a third-year is required to learn, scrawling every possible question in a "history" section, every possible sign in a "physical exam" section, every possible lab I should order with every expected result, surgical options, variant anatomy, mortality and morbidity rates. I was determined not to let this happen to me in the actual combat situation.

Rumors abound about the format of the orals. Everyone's talking about the "good cop-bad cop" routine, where Dr. X's sole goal is to fluster you by acting condescending and boorish, while Dr. Y takes a softer approach, even occasionally chides Dr. X for being such a meanie. It has also been said that students are occasionally asked how stupid they are in the middle of an exam.

One student who came in exceptionally prepared, I am told, was asked the first-line chemotherapy treatment for malignant melanoma. This is something of an unfair question, since almost all melanomas are treated strictly by surgical excision, *not* through chemo. It's a pretty arcane question, especially for a third year. But, being the prepared, honors-level student that he was, he answered correctly. Okay, they said, what's the *second*-line chemo treatment? Even then, he was able to give the correct response. At this point, he's answering a question that may pertain to the treatment of, maybe, on a bright sunny day, a hundred patients in the U.S. They say, very good — now can you tell us the *third*-line chemo regimen?

If I get that kind of a question I'm fried, but I am *not* going to go down without a fight, and I'm going to be able to tell those bastards everything they ever cared to know about thyroid neoplasms, ulcerative colitis, gastric ulcers, cholecystitis, the rule of nines, whatever. Dr. Burn Surgeon made sure of that.

Wednesday, August 23

I left surgery at the VA with a bang. Something like that, anyway. I had figured that, on my last day, I should probably make an effort to actually show up at a surgery, since I had managed to make it to oh, say, five surgeries the entire month. At Christ, I could sit in on three or four every *day*. There was a fem-pop bypass scheduled from 7:30 to 10:30 today—a vascular surgery where a clogged artery in the leg is bypassed by a large, grafted vein. We were supposed to go off-service at noon so that we could have a full day to study for the written exam tomorrow. I figured this was the perfect way to spend the morning, given that the other option was to see the parade of patients in the clinic. Clinic is not a very fun place to be, since the majority of the patients are coming in for routine post-op checks, so one tends to look at incision scars and checks to see if the wound healing is progressing nicely. So one last surgery seemed a good place to be. Finish up before eleven, wander aimlessly for a bit, and then take my leave to go pound the books.

Problem is, I just took my leave from the surgeons a half-hour ago and surgery is *still* going. We made it to 10:30 and it was clear to me that we weren't anywhere near being finished, but I figured we'd make it by noon. Then 11:30 comes around and I'm wondering if I should say anything, thinking it's a *real* bad way to leave your rotation by nagging your doctors about how you want out of the place. I'm still thinking this at 12:30. By 1:30 I've stopped thinking about anything related to the surgery and am, instead, in full-panic mode. Finally, at 2:30, I finally squeaked, in the softest, most sheepish way that a six-foot-two guy with a baritone voice can, if it would be permissible for me to leave so that I could, um, you know, study for tomorrow's Big Test.

Everyone turned and looked at me, as I had been doing little other than stand around for several hours, occasionally retracting. "What time are you supposed to go off service?" they asked. "Noon? Jesus, what are you doing here? Get out of here, man! Go study!"

Which is precisely what I'm about to do.

Thursday, August 24

Orals done, now the written is left.

Two hours ago, I found myself staring into the eyes of Dr. Trendelenberg, one of the senior trauma surgeons. "So, how did you like the past two months?" he started out after he offered me a seat.

"I enjoyed it very much, sir."

"Excellent. Shall we begin? Tell me, what are the most important risk factors for breast cancer?"

He swishes the jump shot! I told him.

"What's the most common type of breast cancer?"

"Infiltrating ductal." C'mon, dude, hit me with a *tough* one!

"What's the survival rate?"

"For what stage?"

"Well, why don't you tell me the criteria for staging, and the survival rates of each stage?"

High inside fastball—but oh my! That's a shot over the right field wall!

I told him.

On to pancreatitis—"What are Ranson's criteria?" Then some questions on colon cancer. Then a scenario of how to evaluate a patient who comes in with a mass on the neck, which turns out to be a thyroid carcinoma. As I answered I thought I was pretty much hitting them on the nail, and I realized how much help it was to be terrified for two solid weeks, even if it did cost me a few Depend undergarments from the intermittent diarrhea.

"Okay, one last question," he says. "What are the common abnormalities found in the MEN II-B syndrome?"

Oh shit. "Well, there's medullary thyroid carcinoma and pheochromocytoma." He stares at me, no expression on his face. I *know* there's something else, but can't remember what.

"Oh, hell," I say. "Cutaneous neoplasms?"

"Mucosal neuromas," he says, and starts to make some notes on the sheet in front of him that displays my name prominently at the top. He stands up, offers his hand, and wishes me luck on the written test.

"Thanks very much, doctor," I said, astonished at how much better this was going than I had anticipated. To even have a shot at honors, I need to get at least in the mid-90s.

two

september in suburbia:

all in the family (medicine)

Monday, August 28

Although I've only gone through orientation, it's difficult to miss the sea change between the surgery and family medicine clerkships. I woke up throughout most of my surgery clerkship at about 5:30; in family medicine, I will be getting up nearly two hours later. During one week of surgery, I could expect to work between 80 and 100 hours, and when not on duty, the attendings expected us to be intensively studying. By contrast, this morning, Dr. Richard, the course director, apologized to us in advance if any of us had to work more than 45 hours in a given week, and said if that happens, he should be consulted immediately. He advised us not to read ahead in the syllabus, but instead to browse through a relevant chapter after we had seen a patient with a given medical issue. I wondered if at some point we were going to receive milk & cookies and be told to take a five-minute nap on our sit-upons.

The change in attitude about work is so dramatic it's tempting to regard family docs and surgeons not as different breeds but as different species, as different from surgeons as kittens are from pirhanas. Not surprisingly, when Richard found out that each of us had just finished surgery, he rolled his eyes. "Well, we do things a little differently around here," he said. True to his word, we finished orientation just past three, about 90 minutes early, and were told to enjoy the rest of the day. Enjoy? What the hell is he talking about?

Monday, September 4

I have been stationed to work with a doctor out in Middletown, Ohio named Ronald Mittleschmerz III, MD. Ronald is in practice with his father, Ronald Mittleschmerz II, who will be retiring at the end of the year. (Yes, there is a Ronald IV.) Taking the place of the elder Mittleschmerz is Laura Williamson, who is fresh out of her family medicine residency. Thus, the practice I'm in is in something of a state of flux.

steven hatch

Middletown is a town of about 40,000 people three-quarters of the way from Cincinnati to Dayton. When I got directions to their office, I was unaware of this distance, assuming it to be a suburb just beyond Cincinnati's outer belt. On Tuesday morning, when I first drove out there, I passed the outer belt and began looking for the exit. I kept looking. No, that's not the right exit, and not that one either. As I kept driving, I think I got a feel for what it must have been like for one of the crewmen on Christopher Columbus's ships: When am I gonna fall off the edge of the earth? At last, mercy, I see the exit for Middletown. I've been on the freeway for 45 minutes, which is the first time in my life that I've actually driven a distance worthy of being called a commute.

Their office is a small, one-story building that makes a poor attempt at being attractive, with a faux-Georgian exterior: A "porch" which is nothing more than a glorified doorway, with cheesy Doric columns and aluminum-siding shutters riveted into the brick. It's awful to look at, but no worse than any of the other developments that line the mile-and-a-half stretch from the highway to his office, which includes large supermarkets or strip-malls with their two-acre-sized parking lots; ubiquitous pizza take-outs; gas stations; convenience stores such as 7-Eleven, Circle K, what have you; trendy new middlebrow restaurants such as The Olive Garden and Don Pablo's; and no sense that there's a center of this vast commercial space. You see, despite its distance from Cincinnati, Middletown is becoming a commuter suburb.

However, the patients coming in to see Drs. Mittleschmerz II & III are, by and large, lifelong Middletonians and have been seeing Dr. Mittleschmerz II when he began practicing here 38 years ago. These patients and their children—and in some cases grandchildren—are still coming back. Because of this family-type atmosphere in the office, many patients aren't put off by the fact that Ronald the Younger frequently runs up to two hours behind. The tradeoff for the patients—and I assume this is why they are willing to put up with such delays—is that they are given ample time to talk about not only their medical problems, but their social circumstances, their marital lives, their children and whatnot. Ronald and Son know their patients very, very well.

The senior Ronald has been practicing in Middletown since he completed his residency. His patients, mostly seniors who began seeing him when he began his practice, are loyal to him. They adore him. They will not see other doctors, and many have been heartbroken by the news of his departure. I followed him around today and it was obvious that he had his shtick down pat. When he was with patients, he was in his element, and the patients knew how to play their appointed role:

"Good afternoon, Doctor!"

He has a broad smile. Even I want to hug him. "Good afternoon, Mrs. Sickalot! I have a student with me here this month, this is Dr. Hatch." He does not pause to gauge whether or not she is comfortable with this. She does not appear to be concerned. "How has your reflux been over the last two months?"

"Oh, doctor," she leans in confidentially, as if giving a stock tip, with a wink in her eye, "you know, that Protonix has just done wonders for me! I'm just thrilled to be using it. I was so tired of having all that pain."

"Gone!" He sort-of states it, but he's asking her a question. She knows this.

"Pretty much."

"Nausea!"

"No, not really."

"Vomiting!"

"All gone."

"Diarrhea! Constipation! Weight loss!"

"No. I feel so much better!"

The rest of the appointment went like this, with him barking-asking questions (though barking isn't the best word, since there's nothing gruff in his voice at all) and Mrs. Sickalot chirpily responding to the battery of questions.

Ronald Three has many of the same qualities as Dad, but obviously he has been trained in a different age, so I believe that he's got a much greater degree of comfort talking about "issues" in medicine that may not have been talked about when his father received his medical training at the University of Cincinnati almost fifty years ago. However he, too, has quite a bit of vanilla flavoring in his recipe mix. At the end of my first day with him, I wanted to ask him how he felt things had gone, whether there was anything in my approach or clinical thinking that he felt he needed to address straightaway. "Oh, no, your clinical acumen seems quite good," he said. "I'm just tickled to have you here."

Um, tickled?

"Dr. Ronald," as the staff calls him to differentiate him from his father "Dr. Mittleschmerz," always allows his patients to complete their sentences. He never cuts them short, even when they've gotten sidetracked from the reason why they came to the office in the first place. At first I thought that he was just an example of a physician who practices medicine in a simple, country manner, and that he had taken his cues from Dear Old Dad. In part, this is true, but I think he is always running two hours late for a much more simple reason: He doesn't know how to say 'no' to his patients, or anyone else for that matter.

Wednesday, September 6

One of the pleasures that must be inherent in doing family medicine is that you're constantly seeing *different* patients as you progress from one appointment to the next. In the two days that I've been back since the Labor Day weekend, I've seen everything from pediatric patients to twenty year-old females needing gynecological care to forty year-old men with headaches to 85 year-olds with breathing troubles. When on Surgery at the VA, I got used to seeing the same patient: He was about 55, he had smoked roughly two packs a day for the last 40 years, he had a heart attack in 1995 and he now has half-dollar sized ulcers on his ankles and feet.

The past two days have been, by contrast, gynecologic, pediatric, and depression days at the office. I've sat in on a few pelvic exams of post-menopausal women, talked to several people about the potential benefits of Prozac, and seen my first case of acute otitis media, the ear infection that plagues infants and toddlers. That variety in patient population seems to me the sole advantage of being a family doc. I can think of several disadvantages.

One of the disadvantages is that you do very little "diagnosing" of serious medical conditions in the office. When a family doc suspects that something serious is going on in a patient, he or she will farm them out to a specialist, who will then order the specific whiz-gidget tests to provide a definitive diagnosis. Then, should a serious disorder be diagnosed, that specialist will either continue to care for them or pass them on to yet other specialists. Only after the acute problem has been resolved will the family doc become involved with the patient's care again, and once again they'll fulfill their role as Primary Prevention Person. There's very little glory in the job.

Another major problem is that they often find themselves seeing patients with recurrent problems, and these patients often don't care for themselves. "I used to think that when I got here, fresh out of residency, I was going to change the world," Dr. Ronald said to me the other day, in reference to one patient whose medical condition is going down the tubes. "I've come to realize that I'm not going to do much more than maintenance for them until they want to change their lives." Thus, much of what Ronald does each day is apply band-aids to wounds but not heal the condition causing the wound—it's not his fault, mind you; he's fully aware of what needs to be done to make a person healthy. But if the patient isn't willing to change, very little of what a doctor does matters much. I guess this is true of any doctor, not just a family doc.

Still, the biggest reservation I have about family medicine is that I can't possibly understand how a doc could manage to do *all* of it well—how someone could keep up with the latest goings-on in internal medicine, pediatrics, gynecology, geriatrics. It seems to me to be just too much to learn. After all, if there is a subspecialty just for pediatric medicine, would you want to send your kid to someone who spent half of residency working with adults?

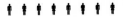

Most of Dr. Ronald's practice consists of geriatric care, since he inherited his father's aging patient base, as well as those of his father's partner, who passed away a few years ago. If I see 15 patients in a day (which is an average number— Ronald will see usually 25 and Dr. Williamson, who after only two months in the practice has not developed a following yet, sees about seven or eight), about ten are over age 50, and the remaining five are split between early middle-aged adults and children less than five. I've seen two or three adolescents, but that age group seems conspicuously absent from this practice. They could well be absent from *all* medical practices, as far as I know. I know that the only time I ever went to a doctor when I was in high school was to get clearance to attend university or play on the baseball team.

What has surprised me thus far is how much I enjoy being with the geriatric patients. They're fun. They like to joke around, they generally don't take themselves or us too seriously, and unless they're in pain, they regard their medical problems as minor nuisances instead of insurmountable obstacles, an attitude I see in some of the younger patients. Most of these patients have the advantage of looking back on a satisfying life, and the family that often accompanies them to the office are testaments to the legacies that they will leave. These people know, for the most part, that they will not be forgotten, that there are loved ones in their life who care deeply about their happiness and how they live out their days, and that they lived mostly a good life about which they can be proud.

I'd be tempted to think that this is the kind of pleasure that a doctor specializing in geriatrics could experience, but something tells me that Ronald's patients are a skewed sample. I wonder how pleasant and upbeat the patients are in many of this nation's nursing homes, the ones who have been forgotten by family members, left to rot away for the last few years of their lives, a burden to be disposed of rather than a resource to be celebrated.

Even in Ronald's practice the scary side of geriatrics creeps in. I was talking to one patient, an 88 year-old woman who was coming in for her yearly checkup. She was entirely pleasant and quite vital; she told me with great pride about the garden that she still tends daily. It was obvious to me that she was in better shape at 88 than either of my grandmothers were at 68. Her heart rate was normal, her lungs were clear and her heart sounded fine. Her blood pressure, however, seemed a little high. It was about 140 over 100. As I was talking to her I looked over her chart, and noticed that she had been diagnosed with borderline hypertension (high blood pressure). Ronald had prescribed her a pill called *Norvasc* that helps keep the blood pressure under control (and thus preventing a host of complications from chronic high blood pressure, the most common and damaging being stroke). I asked her if she was taking her medications.

"Oh no, I don't take them, I haven't for many months," she said. Hmmm, I thought. She didn't look like a patient who wasn't responsible about taking her medications. "You see, my husband has diabetes, and his medications are quite expensive, and we simply can't afford both. So we pay for his medications."

Wednesday, September 13

It's obvious after nearly three weeks in a primary care office that many patients don't enjoy being on meds—well, that's obvious enough. I mean that many of the patients *resist* being on the meds, and I've caught a whiff of resentment directed at the docs as they reach for their scrip pads to assign yet another drug. I get the feeling that Dr. Mittleschmerz and Williamson are caught between a rock and a hard place: They're either drug-happy folks turning a profit for the drug companies by overprescribing, or they're not giving enough care to their patients by underprescribing. And it's often impossible to tell what kind of patient is going to walk into the room: Someone who wants total intervention, or someone who is content to just "watch" a problem until it becomes truly awful.

Plus the fashionable viewpoint at the moment is that doctors overprescribe. Over the past year, there have been many reports about the dire side-effects of "multiple-drug interactions" causing approximately 100,000 deaths each year in the US. This has prompted a great deal of hand-waving among politicians eager to expose the glaring inadequacies of a medical system bent on covering up damaging information like this.

Hear me on this point: It's bullshit. There are, in fact, real problems in the health care system that are being covered up (or at least smoothed over). But one such problem is not doctors who casually overprescribe without considering all of the untoward consequences. The major problem in the health care system is that "the" system is actually several *different* systems and there's a ridiculous amount of bureaucratic waste and inefficiency present, and health consumers are left holding the bag—employers paying the premiums and patients paying the leftovers.

And I don't much doubt that probably something like 100,000 people die from consequences of multiple drug dosing. But what few people understand is that the overwhelming majority of these people are really, really sick, and managing their meds is something akin to walking a tightrope. If they didn't die from the drug interactions, they'd die from heart disease, cancer, or stroke, probably within the same year. And many of them would almost certainly die if they ceased taking *all* their meds. One hundred thousand is an enormous number, but there's also an even larger number of people that are being sustained on meds that are quite tricky to administer, and they're living into their eighties and nineties. But the biggest dirty little secret has nothing to do with careless physicians, greedy drug companies, stingy HMOs and insurance companies, or incompetent hospitals. It's such a simple secret it's almost precious, especially because everyone knows it and no one acknowledges it.

The secret is this: People treat their bodies like shit, and they are fully aware of it, and they don't much care. Once they've harmed their bodies, they come to doctors to get fixed up, which is what doctors do, but very, very imperfectly. The truth is that in many, many instances, people's bodies would work a whole lot better and need doctors a whole lot less if they just treated them better. And doctors tell this to patients every single day. *That's* what becomes plainly evident in three weeks in a family medical practice.

I've been seeing examples of this in lots of patients, but today I found a nearly perfect example of what can only be described as patient stupidity. Linda Percussione is a 56 year-old white female who's been a waitress for well over twenty years. She comes in every six to twelve months for checkups, and she's being followed for recurrent pain in her knees. It could be rheumatoid arthritis, it could be a different form of arthritis, and while it's annoying to her, she has been doing fairly well taking Alleve tablets daily. The problem with taking the daily Alleve, though, has been that she gets an upset stomach (a common side effect of non-steroidal anti-inflammatory drugs, or "NSAIDS" — it's pronounced *en seds* — when used chronically). For that she takes Tagamet, which reduces acid secretion in her stomach.

A few months ago Dr. Mittleschmerz, doing a routine blood check, noticed that she had a high blood glucose, the mark of diabetes, and gave her a talk about the first-line treatment of this kind of diabetes, the late-onset type in adults that we call Type 2 diabetes. The treatment requires no medications, and no invasive or expensive medicine. It *does* require the patient to completely overhaul their diet by eliminating excess calories, working their way down to 1800 calories a day. For people who eat a fair amount — I don't mean gluttons, just people who have a "healthy appetite" — that's a serious restriction. (For instance, a twelve-ounce cola drink has about 150 calories. Drink one at lunch, one for a snack in the afternoon, and one at dinner and you've already used up one-quarter of your day's calories, and you haven't even eaten any actual food. This is not necessarily an outrageous amount of cola to drink, but for a diabetic, that has got to be totally eliminated.)

Ronald sat her down and told her this, that it was going to be difficult, but that it was something she needed to do if she wanted to get better without medications. He proceeded to tell her that the *second* part of this first-line treatment was *exercise*: At least a half-hour of exercise each day in which the patient's heart was beating at about 80 percent of their maximum heart rate, which in this woman's case came out to about 130, give or take. I wasn't there, but I am certain that he conveyed the gravity of the situation, explained the consequences of uncontrolled diabetes which include the kind of ulcers I described while doing surgery, and tried to be as positive as possible about making these lifestyle modifications. He said they would follow-up in a few months, check her blood sugars, and then assess the situation anew.

So when I came to see Linda this morning, her *fasting* blood sugar was 220. That's not as dangerous as the 352 I saw in the patient with the foot ulcer back at the VA, but it's cause for grave concern. Ronald was hoping for her sugars to be in the 100 area. No such luck. While Ronald was with another patient, I talked to her about her blood sugars as well as her other symptoms.

"Well," I said, "How much exercise do you get?"

"Oh, I walk about once a week. For about a half hour."

"Do you have *time* to exercise each night? Like a half-hour or an hour?"

Pause. She's thinking. "Yes, I suppose I do."

"Well, a minimum of a half-hour each day will help keep the sugars in line. Why don't you get that exercise each day?"

"Because I don't *like* to exercise!" she said with some exasperation.

I looked at her. "Well, yes, but you see, that exercise would really help get the sugars under control. It would also help you lose some weight and strengthen your leg muscles, which would probably help a lot with the knees." She wasn't the most obese woman I'd seen but her legs preferentially seemed to like fat on them. If she could lose the weight and increase her strength by walking, it's possible that she'd be able to stop taking the Alleve, which would in turn calm her stomach down, and then no Tagamet.

Instead, she's chosen to ignore the advice that Ronald gave, and now she's not only consigned to these two drugs, but she's going to get put on *another* drug for the diabetes (the next-stop on the treatment journey—after which you try a few other odd drugs, and eventually progress all the way up to insulin injections). When Ronald told her this, she nearly cried. "But I don't *want* to be taking all these medications!" she complained.

The solution? Shut the fuck up, and start walking.

Here's another perfect example of many-patients-don't-really-want-to-listen. Doctors try to prevent death each day cautioning patients about the single most toxic compound known to Americans. To do this, they don't need to do expensive, fancy blood tests to check for mercury or lead levels, and they don't need to reach for their scrip pads to dole out new meds. They don't need to preach the evils of weed, crack, or heroin. They say this: Quit smoking cigarettes. Don't *start* smoking cigarettes. *You'll kill yourself,* and you'll likely die an ugly death on the way.

A lot of people out there aren't getting the message. I'll say it again: Of the major killers in the US—heart disease, cancer, and stroke—only one disease could be virtually eliminated by changing just one simple habit. It will take many different modifications in our lifestyles to reduce the incidence of heart attacks, strokes, or cancers of the colon, prostate, and breast. But stop cigarette consumption and you will have eradicated the biggest killer of all cancers, which clips away at about 150,000 lives per year.

The last patient I saw today was a woman suffering from bronchogenic carcinoma, a particular kind of lung cancer. She's got anywhere from a month to, if she's really lucky, a few years to live. I asked her if she had quit smoking. I did not bother to ask first if she *did* smoke.

"Yes, finally," she responded.

"Good for you," I lied. "When did you quit?"

"Just this year when they diagnosed the cancer," she said. She had had emphysema for years, but was not persuaded to stop despite increasing difficulty with her breathing.

"How many packs of cigarettes did you smoke each day?"

"Three."

"How long did you smoke like that?"

"Since nineteen-forty."

A one-hundred-eighty pack-year history.*

Monday, September 18   7:30 p.m.

I have eaten like a prince for most of my time in Middletown. I have little doubt that, when the bell tolls at the end of my third year, I will have added four to six inches to my waist size from all the free food that drug reps have provided. Drug reps come about four days a week to this inconsequential, *two-doc* practice in little Middletown, and provide lunch, not only to the docs, but the receptionists, the nurses, the secretary, and the med student. It's got to come to about forty bucks a pop every time they do it, and one can assume that if they do it here, then they're feeding the teeming masses of private practice docs everywhere. There's a lotta free food floating around in the medical world, nearly all compliments of drug companies. If you want to lower your food bills, just strap on a white coat and cruise on over to your nearest medical center, find a lunchtime conference, and just stand in line looking like you're supposed to be there.

Admittedly, this practice is something of a hot spot because Dr. Williamson is just getting started, so each rep is courting her like a wildebeest in heat. *I* am becoming familiar with some of these reps, after only three weeks. Apparently the strategy is to bombard Williamson with what amounts to commercials once a week: Say the name "Aciphex" enough, and theoretically she'll reach for her scrip pad and jot down that name for a patient with acid reflux instead of the other

---

* Later in the year, I would discover over in the medicine resident's lounge a board with various medical "records" seen by the residents over the past 15 or so years—like highest blood pressure, lowest heart rate, fastest time from admission to death, and so on. The record for pack-years belonged to a gentleman who, so the report goes, had a—please sit down for this—*440* pack-year history! I find this almost impossible to believe. *Almost* impossible. I could envision some exceptional vets with a can-do attitude who could reach that mark if they could just stay alive long enough.

drugs on the market—Prilosec, Protonix and whatnot. Not that Aciphex is any worse a drug, since they all work at the same molecular level (the so-called 'proton-pump'), but it boils down to brand name loyalty.

Since we're on the subject of slightly morally questionable practices in the health-care industry involving pharmaceutical manufacture, I was talking with Dr. Ronald about how heavily these companies advertise, not only quietly to doctors in situations like these lunches, but quite openly on TV now with commercials. Prescription drugs were never advertised on television until a few years ago, until Congress enacted legislation that allowed pharm companies to do so. So now you see pictures of pretty people running in green fields touting the magic of the new antihistamines (drugs like Allegra, Claritin, or Zyrtec), or of happy people, all smiles, explaining how their lives have changed as a result of taking the newest antidepressants (such as Prozac, Zoloft, and Paxil). The average consumers, at best marginally educated about these drugs and their side effects, see the sheen and think, "yes, that would be good for me!" They proceed to their local docs and ask for scrips.

This is oversimplified, but not jive. "Yeah, it happens more often than you think," Dr. Ronald told me. "Patients will hear about a drug in a commercial, and you will suggest something that will work just as well for them in an over-the-counter form, but they really want the prescription. Like someone with mild acid reflux—there's nothing wrong with the older generation H-two blockers like Zantac, which used to be prescription-only but are now over-the-counter. It's much cheaper to get Zantac than Prilosec, the newer-generation proton-pump inhibitor. But if people see the Prilosec ads and think it's newer and better than Zantac, they'll come in. After all, if they buy the Zantac at the store it's coming out of their pocket, but if I give them a scrip their insurance company pays for it, so they don't see how it costs them and everyone else a little more."

So why not stand your ground and say no?

"Well, sometimes you can coax some patients into trying an older generic or an over-the-counter. But many want what they come for. If I start dictating to my patients what they can or can't do, especially when they're asking for something that's perfectly reasonable, I'm going to risk losing patients, because if they feel like I'm not taking care of their needs, they'll find somebody else who will."

Tuesday, September 19

Surgery grades are back: The first hurdle in the third year race now behind. And I've done well. Very well. I'm pleased as punch to say that I will likely get an Honors in what I thought was going to be the nastiest course of the year.

I got a call from Andrea who told me that they had posted the scores of the oral and written exams outside the Surgery education office, and on the way home from Middletown I dropped by to see the grades. They post the grades with the social security numbers to ensure privacy, but when I looked at the sheet in its entirety the first thing I noticed was one Orals score because it looked longer than the others, like it wasn't placed in the column correctly. When my eye focused on it I saw it was the only *100%* there. Zow, someone must have rocked the boat. My eyes shifted left toward the social security numbers and...no, wait, that *can't* be right. That perfect score belonged to *me*?

After looking at the columns and rows so many times that my eyes nearly bled, I discovered that I had managed the highest score in both the oral *and* the written exam. This morning, I called the department secretary to see if I had it right. "Steven, you did so well on your exams, I'm so proud of you."

The secretary and I had become friendly during the clerkship.

"It's a good thing, too, because I'm so disgusted with your evaluation from Scott," she added.

"What?"

"You know, Scott's evaluation. I couldn't believe what he wrote about you."

"Scott evaluated me?" Scott was one of the senior residents with whom I had few interactions.

"You mean you didn't see it?"

"No, I honestly don't know what you're talking about."

"You'd better drop by today and take a look."

Since I came after-hours, she left me an envelope of this evaluation, which must have come late in the game since I had seen my first two evaluations at Christ. Scott—the senior resident on the Chirst surgery team—very nearly *failed* me, giving me a grade only two points into the passing range. His comments at the bottom included such gems as "does not have good patient rapport...fails to take initiative...unimpressive in nearly all aspects."

Guess I can't make everyone happy. Forgive the hubris, but I'm inclined to dismiss much of these comments as that of a silly ninny who never paid much attention to me. *But...*that's the feeling of someone who crossed the finish line toward the head of the pack. Scott's evaluation didn't drop my final grade to a high-pass, but a point here and a point there on some of the other evaluations or the tests, and my Honors grade is gone. It was a little spooky to realize that I was very nearly at his mercy. I'm only going to be willing to believe that he had a point if I see observations that match his in the coming months. Otherwise, I'm going to assume it was sour grapes—and after seeing the evil bastards in that department and what they do to their residents, I have little doubt that he had been essentially conditioned to be that way.

† † † † † † †

Speaking of grades, I am coming up on a test to complete this course on Friday. I have not studied a drop for it. One of my classmates who had taken it earlier in the summer said it was a waste of time to bother studying for it. I took that as my cue and have focused on my writing and my jump shot in the meantime.

We also are required to write a five-page paper about a particular patient and focus on all the non-medical factors involved with their long-term medical care, such as churches, their work conditions, family members that provide or need care, etc. I've put slightly more time into this, but I'm not sweating this terribly. I *can* write a sentence with a subject and a verb in it, after all, and while I might not be Dostoyevsky, I can certainly compose with more talent than the majority of my over-scienced classmates. I figure even if I make a mistake here or there I've got to look better by comparison.

Thursday, September 21 6:00 p.m.

One more test, and Family Medicine is behind me. I left Middletown in what nearly amounted to a teary-eyed goodbye with the staff and the docs. Because they only have one student a year come through their place, medical students are a special commodity there, something of a break from the day-in day-out tedium that comes with seeing twenty-five patients a day, many of them patients they see on a weekly or monthly basis. I provided different scenery for them, and since we got on well, saying goodbye actually felt like it meant something. It was certainly a different experience from my last day of Surgery.

Though I tried to keep as open a mind as possible for someone who has strong opinions, I knew that Family Medicine was not a specialty for me. I've got some problems with the entire *concept* of family medicine, but we'll deal with that in a moment.

First, in terms of my own professional goals, it appears that being a Family Medicine doc requires seeing *lots* of patients, in and out, boom-boom-boom, every single day. It did not strike me as being any more glorious than my desk job as a science writer before I came to medical school. Not that I didn't like that job, but it felt like just that—a job—something that you do mostly for the purpose of making money to pursue more interesting things in life. That's not really why I went to medical school. Call me naïve or a dreamer, but I think I'm seeking something more akin to a *calling* than a job, something that I think about as my purpose in life rather than my occupation.

Family Medicine, being the most general of medical

specialties, also doesn't really aim to ask deep questions about how the body works. It's perhaps the most practical-minded specialty of all, since its aim (as far as I was able to surmise) is to train private-practice family docs. Oh, I'm sure there's *some* kind of research out there going on in some Family Medicine departments, but my guess is they're of the social-science variety: How much better is a certain type of patient-education program about weight loss in Type II diabetics than another; or, does family counseling about heart disease have better outcomes for patients than cases in which patients are just taught about their conditions by themselves, without any other family members present? These are interesting questions, I guess, but they don't interest *me* a great deal. I'm beginning to think that I'm going to have to find something in which I'm trying to learn, at some basic level, how the body works — and *not* how to make things better for patients. That is a noble pursuit, just not the one that I feel compelled to join.

But like I said, after a month I'm a bit weary of the whole idea of Family Medicine. Family Medicine involves practicing three major subspecialties — Pediatrics, Internal Medicine, and basic Gynecology (Family docs need a one-year fellowship in order to perform basic Obstetric procedures such as delivering healthy babies). Taken separately, it would take *ten years* to train in those specialties! Family docs, though, have only *three*-year residencies. And many of them are not considered to be the most rigorous of experiences.

The justification for these skewed numbers is that Family Medicine is a primary-care driven specialty, with emphasis on the "primary." Docs that perceive something as wacky, such as an abnormal EKG for someone with heart palpitations, send their patients to the hospital or to a cardiologist's office, to be evaluated by a second-layer of more refined expertise.

I have no problem with the idea of primary care, but when you require primary care for such wide age ranges as that seen in Family Medicine, I don't care how hard you work or how smart you are, you are *bound* to miss some of the more subtle presenting complaints of your patients. The idea of see-trouble-and-refer only works if you see the trouble. And though I'm not anywhere close to knowing the specifics, it seems to me that there could easily be a situation where a Family doc might be inclined to blow off, say, fatigue in a fifty year-old guy who says he's been "working real hard lately" while an internist might have a longer list of conditions about which he or she is suspicious. I just can't see how you can do it all and do it well.

three

shrinkage

Monday, September 25

We began the Psych experience by having an orientation at 7 a.m. This put me in a *very* chipper mood. At least the "orientation" lasted only an hour and we were on the wards by 8:15, thus saving us a full day of the "Welcome to…." lectures that the students are basically capable of writing at this point. Each time we start a new rotation we receive such pieces of wisdom as, "it is important that you dress professionally," and "it is considered bad form if you act eager to leave in the afternoons." Someone needs to *explain* this to us? And for the third time in four months?

I'm on the 8th floor East wing lock-down ward for the next three weeks, then have a three-week tour over at Children's Hospital working the inpatient child psych unit; and throughout this six-week period I'll spend every Tuesday afternoon at the Hamilton County Jail "Court Clinic."

The 8 East ward is officially known as the "psychobiology research unit," which means that they're doing drug trials in patients there. I'm not going to be involved with that work. In fact, I'm doing pretty much what every other student is doing everywhere else: Following manic, schizophrenic, and suicidal patients.

There's a quasi-technical word the staff appears to have for some of the patients: *Nuts*. In the morning rounds they'll sit around using fairly jargony language to talk about a patient, like the nurse said about one gentleman today: *He demonstrated no homicidal or suicidal ideation; his auditory hallucinations tend to get worse in the evenings, and he continues to express flight of ideas and disordered thinking.* After she recited this description without any emotion at all, she paused, looked carefully at the attending, and added, "he's nuts."

I'm obviously a beginner at this sort of thing, but I'm gathering that not just any old psych inpatient assumes the title of *nuts*. (Incidentally, *crazy* is also used, but not as much. *Nuts* seems to be the preferred term.) It's a special designation. It means something like this: If you're on the ward, and your medications are keeping you pretty well controlled, you have a *mental illness*. If you're not taking your medications, sleep two hours each night, smell so fetid that even farm livestock would blush, and try to deliver messages from God to the other patients, well then you're *nuts*. Oh, I forgot the most important part: You're nuts when you don't know why the hell you're there in the first place.

The staff laugh a lot about their patients during the morning conference. I think they laugh because, first, it helps them maintain some kind of sanity in what is literally a maddening work environment, and second, some of the things that the patients say are funny. One of the patients had come up to one of the residents, and tapped him on the shoulder this morning. Looking at him earnestly, the patient said, in solemn tones, "I know you think my voice is sexy, but *I* don't." The patient, who had offered up this analysis without further elaboration, had left, apparently satisfied he made his point.

I was assigned to this resident, Dr. Jason Bartholomew, showing once again that God has been merciful to me. Jason, at first glance, appears to be mellow, funny, interested in my education, and willing to take time with me. My classmate working with me on 8 East is not as lucky. Bryant has been assigned to work with Dr. Mustaffa. An Indian immigrant and likely a foreign medical graduate, Dr. Mustaffa seems from my brief meeting with him to be quite cordial. But his accent is thick, and you have to ask him to repeat nearly half of what he says. Also, because he is an immigrant, he's got to have a harder time interpreting the cultural meaning of his patients' circumstances. It's hard enough for the average American-born medical student to deal with these kinds of patients, but the difficulties that he must face with his patients — several of whom must be annoyed by his nationality, no doubt — is almost unimaginable.

I'm also not sure if he's a great physician. When Bryant and I left the lock-down this afternoon, we were accompanied by one of the staff social workers, who had to run an errand. Once he was beyond the range of the unit, he gave us his view of the ward. "You know how they talk about separating the wheat from the chaff? Well, *you* got the wheat," he directs a finger at me, "and *you* got the chaff. Sorry about that, Bryant, but the attending is going to be relying on you for a lot of stuff."

It's not uncommon for foreign medical graduates to try to obtain a residency in the United States so they may be licensed here and thus emigrate. Doctors in the States, even those poorly compensated, earn a handsome salary compared to their counterparts almost everywhere else. Because of this, tens of thousands of physicians trained in institutions outside the US apply for residencies each year. Most have no chance, but the better ones often can secure a residency in programs that simply aren't attractive to home-grown medical students. Both rural residencies and psychiatry programs are frequently short of the resident manpower needed to keep their wards well run, since fewer and fewer American grads choose a career in psych, whose star has long since faded from prominence in the medical field.* That's how a guy like Dr. Mustaffa finds his way in. Some of these foreign medical grads turn out to be worth their weight in gold, and others turn out to be a terrible liability.

Ψ Ψ Ψ Ψ Ψ Ψ Ψ Ψ Ψ

I have been assigned two patients, at least one of whom is *nuts* by the staff's loose definition. Both patients may actually be *nuts*, but I haven't figured out whether the second is included in such elite company. William is the former patient. He came in last Friday, and when I met him today, he wanted to explain to me that he was there to help me with Elizabeth,

---

* And many psych programs also find themselves picking American candidates that appear less than ideal. The most notorious case involves Dr. Michael Swango, who graduated from Southern Illinois University School of Medicine, and thereafter began a poisoning spree that resulted in his arrest, conviction, and imprisonment. After serving two years, he began seeking out residencies again, targeting those two desperate groups mentioned above — rural residencies and psych programs. He worked for a time in an Emergency Medicine program in North Dakota, and several years later he was arrested again in New York working as a Psychiatric resident. For more details, see the book *Blind Eye* by James Stewart.

my other assigned patient. "I am going to be a social worker," he confided to me with wide eyes. His breath reeked of vomit, and the first whiff caught me off-guard, nearly making me wretch. "I am very good with the patients." So why did you come here, I asked. "Oh, to do just what you're doing. To help the patients."

William is an unusual psych patient. He's 42 years old, and this is his first psychiatric hospitalization ever, so far as the staff can tell. His tentative diagnosis is mania, but he might instead have "bipolar disorder," also called manic depression, since he's admitted to prior episodes of depression. Most manics or patients with bipolar do not get hospitalized for the first time at age 42. Like schizophrenia, it's a younger persons disease, typically happening in the late teens and twenties. It's quite possible that he has been cycling through mania and depression for years, but that he has managed to stay functional throughout the previous episodes, and that people may have forgiven his eccentric behavior during such periods. Somehow, he has managed to make it through five decades without a severe manic episode, and he's got a wife, four children, and a job at the local post office. Not doing social work, though.

William is about two feet away from me as he's talking, and I'm not so much bothered by my personal space being invaded as I am by the smell of his breath. "Pick a word, c'mon now, just pick any word," he tells me. I had been told about this earlier in the morning. He wants to show me his ability to "contextualize." The staff was having a hoot when they were describing how William "contexualizes," because what he believes is his almost preternatural skill is what anyone else would call "using a word in a sentence." So I am going to see what he is capable of. I pick a word.

"Baseball."

Shock. "Baseball? Oh, c'mon now, I *know* you can do better than that. Don't just pick any old word, pick a *good* word, pick a *tough* word."

"Okay. 'Psychological.'"

"Allright," he says. He steps back—thank God—and throws his arms out. "Baseball may be 'psychological,' but that's not what's important in the game." He stops, surveys the sentence that he has just spoken, and appears thoroughly satisfied. "You see? That's my gift, and God gave it to me. I can just *do* that with *any* word. God has also allowed me to see the mantle above people — yes, I can just see their mantles. And you may not believe in God, but I'll tell you this, if you do believe in God, your heart will be pure."

It is hard to listen to this without cracking up.

This whole interaction with William occurred after my first meeting with Elizabeth, a 55 year-old woman with schizophrenia. I learned Elizabeth was my patient only after I saw her haranguing Artrell, one of the social workers. "Give me liberty, or give me death!" she was bellowing at him. She was loud, and I wondered if anyone was going to jump to restrain her, but no one appeared concerned. "GIVE ME LIBERTY, OR GIVE ME DEATH!" she repeated, glaring at poor Artrell. "Patrick Henry!" she shouted. No verb followed. Then she marched off to the television room.

"You can see what they're like," Artrell said to me after he entered the resident room.

"Hey, she got the quote right," I said. "She might be psychotic, but she knows her history."

I didn't understand what had caused the outburst, but after I came over to talk to her it became clear: Once she left lock-down she was going to be discharged to a nursing home of some kind, in all likelihood. Before she was admitted to the ward she had been living on her own; now she was being forced into a living arrangement that curtailed her freedom. I was listening to her talk for about ten minutes about how upset she was, basically how *pissed* she was about having to move into a nursing home. She answered all my questions directly, but she never looked directly at me. As I listened, I thought: Where's the *nuts* here? She's upset about having to move out of her home where she maintained independence. What's so unusual about that?

"But why are you so upset about having to move into the nursing home?" I asked. "What's wrong with it?" Then she looked right at me. I had struck a geyser.

"*You* know just what they do, you *doctor*. You think I don't know. I know that you *plastic surgeons* want to cut me up! Just like you cut up my tongue! Just like you cut up that little fourteen year-old colored girl! Ha ha! Ha!"

"So you think that there are doctors that are going to cut you up?" I asked.

"Have you been listening to what I just said?" she shot back. Guess I deserved that. "I know that you have that big, large green button that will make that *radar love voodoo* of yours."

I wasn't sure I heard that right. Was she making a reference to the song "Radar Love" by the long-since defunct band *Golden Earring*? "I'm sorry, but what was the button?" I asked.

Same glare as before, like the *are you stupid, Steven?* look I got from several surgeons back in the summer. "You think you're going to give me that radar love voodoo! You think that you'll be able to press that button and just make me feel that radar love voodoo and make me do things with other women! No! Ha ha! Ha! I'm not going to let you do that to me! None of that radar love voodoo! No!"

It is hard to listen to this without cracking up.

Friday, September 29

It was a rough week for our man William. We had enrolled him in a drug trial testing a new medication for "mood stabilization." When a patient enrolls in a drug trial, we explain to them the possible side effects, the fact that this is a test using human subjects, that they are in effect "guinea pigs" although safety trials have already been performed. We also explain to them that the trial is what is known as a "double-blind placebo-controlled" trial, which means that some patients are given the real medication while others are given a "fake" pill (or placebo). When the physicians and nurses administer the meds, they do not know which patients are assigned the real medication and which are assigned placebos, nor do the patients (thus *double*-blind). That said, we knew that William was in the placebo group.

Now we're not "supposed" to know this, and we do not

know with total certainty whether he was actually in the placebo group. But after the first 24 hours he took the trial drug, he got worse. Much worse. First, he had come up to a new patient and fondled her breasts, apparently while espousing his religious beliefs. This woman, who is another one of "my" patients, apparently did not find the behavior entirely objectionable.

Then he paced the halls on Tuesday night the *entire* night, walking into other patients rooms, asking if he could pray with them, praying on his own when others decided to opt out of 3 a.m. prayers, and possibly intruding into other patients, um, private spaces, let's call it. None of the staff witnessed any particular incident but another patient, Mr. Gosselin (who is likely on the ward because he doesn't want to be in jail, not because he's actually ill) started screaming that he was going to kill William because "I saw that motherfucker sucking on that guy's dick!" — referring to his roommate whom William came to bother during the night. It escalated to a fight, and the staff had to break up the scuffle. When we arrived Wednesday morning, one of the nurses looked at me when I said "good morning," and said, "I have been working in psych wards for over ten years, and this has been the worst night of my career."

That Wednesday morning we gave him enough Ativan to kill a large horse, but it didn't slow him down a bit. Meanwhile, his wife had learned from their pastor, who had dropped by to visit, that he hadn't been improving, and she called up to insist that it was time to get him off the trial drug and onto some *real* meds. Dr. Nesterovich had urged her to stay the course for 24 more hours, but she wouldn't hear of it. From the standpoint of medical science, we wanted him on just a bit longer to make the data for the study as pure as possible — the longer you follow out a patient and show a change in behavior (with meds) or lack thereof (without), the better case you can make that the medication works. From the standpoint of the sanity of the staff and the other patients, getting William off the study and onto other meds was like manna from heaven.

It took a solid day but we finally got him calmed down, and by this morning he was almost looking like a normal human being again—a religious freak human being, mind you, but a human being nonetheless. After the weekend, William was ready for discharge.

Ψ Ψ Ψ Ψ Ψ Ψ Ψ Ψ Ψ

DeShante is not my patient, and I don't know what's wrong with her, even though it looks like mania to my untrained eye. She acts a bit like William. She'll pace the hallway, sing out religious verses in the shower, and walk in and out of patient rooms no matter the time of day. One night she had become quite agitated (this was Tuesday night, the same night that William was at the peak of his disruptive energies), and ripped all the privacy curtains that separate one patient's "space" from another's, screaming bloody murder all the way. Finally, when the staff could take it no more, she was placed in the "stimulation reduction room," which is a lockdown within the lockdown, similar to the padded room of popular imagination.

When I came in Wednesday morning, DeShante was standing in the doorway of the seclusion bay, from the inside looking out. She was marching in place, and even though you could only see her from her chest up, you could count her paces just from watching her head bob up and down. When staff walked by they would look in, and she would point at them. Not missing a beat, they'd point back, and go about their business.

When my classmate Andrea came by to grab me to go to lunch, she looked in at DeShante and asked what she was doing in there. I explained, and suggested as we were walking out that she wave hello. Andrea did, and DeShante waved right back, her head still bobbing up and down.

Ψ Ψ Ψ Ψ Ψ Ψ Ψ Ψ Ψ

I have two new patients on my roster. One, Linda Minor, is a mother of a four year-old, whom she loves very much. She was living on her own in Idaho for many years, but began traveling the West in a camper because she believed that someone was spying on her. She also believed that her parents were in a Satanist cult, and with the help of the US government, had placed an implant in her brain. Her last stop was North Dakota, and when she arrived in Bismarck, she called the police several times about the spies, and eventually, the police decided it was time to take her in for psychiatric help.

This woman would likely still be in a psychiatric hospital in Bismarck were it not for the efforts of her mother, who refused to allow her grandchild to move into a permanent foster care home. She learned that the only way to get her grandchild out of the system was to work at getting her daughter out. I'm not clear on the details but it seems the hospital was willing to release Ms. Minor to her mother. The three of them came back to Cincinnati about one month ago, with Linda promising the whole way home that she was going to take medication and seek help. Upon returning to Cincinnati, she did neither, tucking herself away in a local motel. Her mother, fearing for the child, finally called the police to help out. She was admitted to Psychiatric Emergency Services, who placed a "hold" on her, meaning that she would be admitted to the hospital involuntarily for 72 hours. During that time, the mother was granted temporary custody of the child, and there's a hearing scheduled for a continuation of that temporary custody next Friday.

The thing that struck me when I first came to see Linda Minor was how unusually *normal* she looked. A woman in her early forties, she was quite pretty, which my resident even noted in his admission history: "41 year-old white female, attractive, with five-year history of bipolar disorder...." She was well groomed, which many of the patients aren't. Even when you talked to her, you didn't get the sense that anything was wrong. Initially. Unlike William, Ms. Minor didn't sing out her psychoses, didn't have the "psycho eyes" that are so plainly visible on other patients. But about five minutes of conversation made clear her problems.

Not only does she believe that there were spies watching her, not only does she believe that her family are Satanists placing things in her brain (she even invited me to see the "scar" on her head where they inserted it—and of course there was nothing there), but she is extremely preoccupied with the subject of rape. She doesn't claim to have been raped (except possibly as a child, but the story and the identity of the rapist often change), but her preoccupation with the subject has filtered down to her daughter. When the grandmother got custody, one of the social workers working for the county came out to visit her to establish if her mother had put her in any harm. It became pretty clear that there was a lot of talk about rape, and that the child was quite concerned about being raped, but didn't actually know what constituted "rape."

It was also clear that she focused much of her paranoia on all of her family members. You would think that if someone had managed to survive a childhood in a cult that all they would want to do is get away from them and never speak to them again. But Ms. Minor was in constant contact with the family, writing regularly to her brother and frequently calling her mother. I had even seen a recent picture of Linda, her daughter, and her mother when they were in North Dakota. They all look perfectly happy together.

With William and Elizabeth, this loco behavior is cute in its own very sad way. With Ms. Minor it's only sad. I don't know what's going to become of the custody issue, but I think there are two major possibilities. One is that Ms. Minor will refuse to acknowledge that there's a problem, will resist treatment and medications, and will thus manage to lose custody of her child. For instance, she might be released from the hospital, and immediately proceed to her mother's house and demand that her daughter come with her. That will precipitate a call to the police, and once they get involved, she's going to end up in the psych ward again, and if it happens enough, the grandmother's going to get permanent custody.

But I'm betting on another outcome after having talked to Ms. Minor for a few hours. Any woman who can raise a child on her own with a serious mental disturbance, and do it on about one thousand dollars a month (she collects her father's social security, a benefit she figured out from doing careful research), is a very intelligent woman. Her mother told us that despite the low annual income (she doesn't work), the child seems to have been well provided for. My guess is a woman capable of *that* is capable of rationally figuring out how to get out of the hospital with her doctor's blessings, how to convince her mother and a judge that she has improved and is fit to have custody returned. Once her daughter is back with her, she will slip out of Dodge very quietly.

Ψ Ψ Ψ Ψ Ψ Ψ Ψ Ψ Ψ

The other new patient is Missy Salina, age 31. Like Ms. Minor, she has a chronic bipolar disorder. Unlike Ms. Minor, she's not able to function very well in the outside world. She was living in California when she called her mother to come for help, because she said she was going "to get a gun and end it all." It was a threat that the mother took quite seriously, and she came, brought her back, and after a quick trip through psych emergency services, she landed up on 8 East on the same 72 hour hold that has Ms. Minor in our custody.

Missy Salina is younger than Linda Minor but she looks like life has beat her up a good deal more. She's unkempt, her clothes are dirty, she's morbidly obese, and her eyes have a terrible sunken look. I wonder what she looked like when she was in high school. Her family lives in Wyoming, one of the more exclusive suburbs of metropolitan Cincinnati, and she attended an exclusive prep school during her high school years. I can't imagine her at that prep school with her current appearance. She alleges that part of the reason for her current sorry state is a severely traumatic event involving a back-alley abortion and an abusive boyfriend. The back-alley part sounds like jive to me but her mother confirms the story — or at least says that *she* believes it's true. At any rate, the trauma causes her to become extremely agitated: She insists that she is "upset" because of that and not any psychiatric problems, and we're not going to be able to help her with this problem. I'm thinking that every minute of her time with us is going to be spent locked in battle, with her resisting our every effort.

Tuesday, October 3

Things haven't been going well with my patients. I have stopped formally following Elizabeth's care since I picked up the caseload for Ms. Minor and Ms. Salina. That's a pity, too: I don't get to hear any more "radar love voodoo" type remarks. (The last time I spoke with her at length she told me that she was bothered by the "screwdriver bugs" in her hair. I'll miss remarks like that.) Ms. Minor no longer wants to talk to me, and Ms. Salina has spent virtually every minute of her time ranting about how she wants to get out, immediately, that she's perfectly fine and can take care of herself.

She's not, of course. If we let her out today or tomorrow, she would bolt for California as soon as it was feasible. She wouldn't take her meds, and she'd sink right back into the same hole that sent her calling her mother in the first place. And her behavior on the ward shows that she's not improving at all. Yesterday she came up to me and told me that her mother was demanding to come and pick her up. She had just gotten off the phone with her, and her mother was extremely disappointed with us. Since we had a changeover of residents (Jason, like most residents, rotates through sites just as we students do; Dr. Nesterovich, the attending physician, is on a one-week vacation), I was the only person around familiar enough to talk with her mother, so I fielded her phone call.

"Missy tells me that you think she's ready to be discharged," she said. "I was kind of surprised by this, but she seems really unhappy there. Do you think that she would benefit from leaving?"

"Well, ma'am, I first want to explain to you that I'm only a medical student, and I can't make any binding decisions in terms of her care, so let's be clear on that," I said. She told me we were clear. "That said, I think I'm speaking for the staff when I say that we do *not* believe that she's ready to be discharged. Our plan for her that we discussed with her last Thursday, when she signed the voluntary admission, is that she would need about ten days to get her stabilized, and we were targeting Monday October 9th as her discharge day. I was there when we discussed this with her and I'm certain that we made that quite clear to her."

"Oh. I didn't know that she was aware of that." Naturally. After I got off the phone with her mother, I came back in to tell her that we were going to stay the course (which I had convinced her mother was the best way to proceed) and that we were looking at next Monday as a target date. I also added that I wanted to do anything I could to help her make her time here go as smoothly as possible. She screamed at me for about ten minutes. It wasn't the most pleasant ten minutes of the day, but I knew that I had handled the matter correctly despite not checking with my new resident or attending.

Ψ Ψ Ψ Ψ Ψ Ψ Ψ Ψ Ψ

Meanwhile, Ms. Minor continues to believe that she's being held here by her parents so that they can steal custody of her daughter from her, that there's nothing at all wrong with her (sound familiar?), and that she doesn't need to even be *taking* her medications, but she especially doesn't need to be taking *new* medications.

That's where everything went sour. Dr. Darvon is the attending who's sitting in while Dr. Nesterovich is gone. At the Monday morning meeting (in which we review the patients' conditions and change any plans for the patients' care if need be), Dr. Darvon decided that Ms. Minor needed to be on another medication called *Trilafon*, a strong antipsychotic. He hadn't met her yet, and when he suggested it to Jason, I glanced at him to read his reaction. Jason didn't openly disagree, but I knew that he had misgivings about it. We had struggled for three days just to get Ms. Minor to *increase* her level of Zyprexa (another antipsychotic). We felt pretty good about getting her to agree to that, but it wasn't easy.

Now we were going to tell her that we were going to add another medication to her regimen, and I knew that she wasn't going to buy it. This is a woman who thinks that someone has been putting implants in her head and that people are spying on her. How open is she going to be to take another little pill each day from people who have locked her up? What upset me was that Jason didn't object to adding the new med. "Hey, why'd you let Darvon add that prescription? She's your patient, tell him that it's not a good idea."

"You crazy, man? Listen, I know that shit runs downhill, and I'm just one stop along the way," he said. "I don't make the decisions, I just implement them."

It was a disaster. Jason ran into her in the hallway on the ward, and he tried to explain to her that they wanted her to add another med. She balked immediately, saying that she was doing just fine. "No, you're not doing fine, Ms. Minor. You've had a chronic mental disease for at least five years that's gone untreated, and things are not going to get better overnight. Taking these meds will help you along that way, but you're still paranoid, you're distrustful, and your thoughts are still racing."

That didn't go over so well. Of course, Jason left that afternoon to go on to the VA for his next rotation. I don't fault him for that, but he didn't have to deal with the fallout. I did. When I came up to her later in the day, I asked her if it was okay for us to talk.

"You know, I've been wanting to tell you something about that," she said. "I don't want to talk to you anymore. I mean, you're very nice, and I've been talking to you like you're a friend, but you're a student, and you're not here to do anything for *me*, isn't that right? And now, the doctors are thinking that I'm *crazy* and I'm wondering 'Why does everyone think I'm crazy?' And then I realize that I've been talking to *you*. And all you've been doing is just listening to me, you've just been taking things in, and you haven't told me anything, have you? Well, I think that you've been going around telling these people that I'm crazy."

"Wait a minute. Hold on. I want you to understand that yes, I'm here as a student, but I'm also here to help you out in any way I can."

"But how can you do that? I want some real help. I want a psychological," she told me. I think by 'psychological' she meant some formal testing. "I just need someone to give me a psychological and tell me that everything's fine so that I can go back and get my daughter. In the meantime, I really don't want to talk to you. I mean, don't take it personally. I think you're really cute, but I just don't feel comfortable talking to you anymore." And with that, she walked away. I haven't talked to her since, except when I came up to her in the hallway this morning and asked her if she had changed her mind. "No, I don't want to, but that's a *really* nice tie," she said.

Ψ Ψ Ψ Ψ Ψ Ψ Ψ Ψ Ψ

William has left the psych unit. Though still very odd, he is remarkably more subdued than he was upon entry. He wanted to leave us a token of his stay here, and he produced the following poem (without editorial changes or spelling corrections):

Help on Ward 8
Ward Eight will always have a special place in my heart.♥
Because it set my mind from evil thoughts.
Once my mind was held captive.
However now it is free as a bird
Able to soar new hights to the unknown.

Now I know my mind isn't broken.
And it sharper day by day.
Thanks for giving me the answer to unclearness
In my mind
Now I able to face the expected with courage
And respect instead of fear.

Wednesday, October 4

Missy Salina's drama of the day was another misunderstanding between her mother and her. She wanted to know if I would intervene and again petition for her to go to California. I asked what had gone on with her mother, and, in tears, she explained that her mother is a major force of evil in her life and would I please talk to her. I said that I was planning to call just to see what was going on in terms of arranging another meeting at the end of the week.

"Oh, that's *so* wonderful, thank you so much," she said. "You know, you're the only person around here that's been listening to me. You're the only one that understands what's really going on."

"Uh, sure. Well, we'll see how things go after I talk to your mom." Was this really the same person who had said, less than forty-eight hours ago, I was a "stupid motherfucker" who wanted to torture her? Amazing.

Thursday, October 5

Ms. Minor explained to the social worker, Artrell, yesterday that the reason why she didn't want to talk to me had little to do with not trusting me, it had to do with her "sexual feelings" for me. She said that her attraction to me interferes with her ability to talk with me. So I've essentially dropped her from my "care" list. That, coupled with William's discharge on Monday, means that all I've got is Missy Salina.

We had a meeting this morning between Missy, her mother, her aunt, Dr. Stratford (my new resident), Artrell, and me. It got us nowhere. Missy is going back to California as soon as she's out, and she really doesn't want to hear anything else that anyone has to say. To appease her mother, she said that her "plan" was that she would go back, put her house on the market, and move back to Northern Kentucky and get a job here in the greater Cincinnati area. But wait, her mother replied, why not look for an apartment in Northern Kentucky *now* if you plan to move anyway? No, no, I just want to get back to California, she answered. Meaning: I'm not *really* planning to move back to this area, but I don't want this to turn ugly, so just play along with me.

I doubt I'm going to have much else to say about her until she's discharged next Monday. She'll leave, and she'll head back to California. She might get follow-up care, but my guess is that she'll eventually stop taking her medications, and with nobody there for her, she's going to fall back into a hole. It's possible that she'll commit suicide. This isn't just my uneducated appraisal: The nursing staff, the social worker, and my resident all concur that this is in her future.

Wednesday, October 11

For the educational portion of the course, instead of having traditional lectures, the course director Dr. Barnett has created a "case conference" setup. The students are given a clinical vignette about a common psychiatric condition, and there is a list of reading assignments on the following page that are to be read before the case conference. Four or five students are assigned to serve as "experts" on those articles and answer questions posed by the professor or classmates, and each session lasts about two hours.

Most people who aren't the "experts" don't do the assigned reading, and the more clever students arrive early enough to sit in strategic positions in the conference room so that they can rest their heads with a minimum level of detection by the shrink-du-jour. Fortunately, studying for psych isn't quite as rigorous as studying for medicine or surgery, so people who haven't done the assigned reading can fake it, and don't appear to be completely stupid.

Hearing stories from the shrinks during these sessions helps even more to solidify what we're learning in the wards. Anorexia nervosa is an easy enough disease to recognize, and it's equally easy to remember that it's one of the most lethal psychiatric conditions, since the patients starve themselves to death. But how do they die? It's not a mere matter of losing weight until they waste away. The answer is that the body's electrolytes are thrown into such wild fluctuations that the heart, which needs to maintain a delicate electrolyte balance to function, can generate fatal arrhythmias. They die of heart attacks.

This, by itself, is a tough piece of information to digest simply because there's no hook to hang it on in one's brain. Isolated, it doesn't seem so bad, but you have to remember *hundreds* of little facts like these to be competent. During one of these sessions an attending, Dr. Frekko, was describing his experience with an anorexic who routinely purged (not all anorexics vomit to maintain low weight; most just starve). She had been through the hospital so many times that she had become quite sophisticated in her understanding of the biochemistry of her body, and knew what doctors were worried about in relation to her heart — namely that dramatic swings in the amount of potassium could stop her heart, and potassium decreases after vomiting.

"I was a resident, working on the wards, and I was discussing her case with her one morning. She said she could control her potassium even better than she could control her weight. I asked her what she meant. She said, 'Doc, what's my potassium level?' and I told her it was 4.2."

A "normal" level of potassium is between about 3.5 and 5.1.

"She said, 'Okay, now go get somebody to draw my blood, and watch this.' She didn't even have to put her finger in her mouth; she could just spontaneously induce vomiting. Later, when we drew her blood, her potassium went down to two-point-eight."

Now *that's* a piece of information to hang the other stuff on.

Today's topic was personality disorders, and borderline personality disorder was being discussed extensively. Many personality disorders do not come to the attention of psychiatrists because they actively *avoid* doctors and hospitals, but patients with borderline personality disorder, who often attempt suicide many times, are disproportionately seen in psychiatry practices.

"Nobody really knows what causes it, but one of the popular theories is that borderline personality disorder starts in early infancy, when baby is with mother and all is happy — the baby thinks of the world as being 'everything good with me and mommy' and 'everything bad and scary outside of me and mommy,'" said Dr. Frekko, who was leading the class that day. "But the next phase of development, where baby recognizes that it is a separate and autonomous individual from mommy, fails to happen. So that person spends their whole life trying to get back to that Garden of Eden where everything is happy.

"They'll find a person, and if they like them they'll cling very tightly to them, and that person can't do any wrong, they're the best person in the world, they're perfect, just like mommy was. But the moment when conflict arises -- and all relationships have conflict, which is what healthy adults cope with on a daily basis — between someone with BPD and the idealized other, that person suddenly is thrown back out into the 'outside me and mommy' realm, and the person sets about in search of another to fill the role. People can go in and out of the 'mommy' role — it's not a permanent exile — and relationships with these people can be rocky indeed."

Her "official" diagnosis is bipolar disorder, but that's as perfect a description of Missy Salina as I can think of.

Saturday, October 14

Missy Salina was discharged last Tuesday and has "decided" to remain in the Cinicnnati metro area. I don't know the details, but my guess, and it's a good one, is that her father was notified of the meeting by Missy's mom, and he laid his foot down. Since he has held the purse strings, paying not only the mortgage of the California home but $450 in monthly expenses as well, Missy wasn't in much of a position to negotiate. She was able to play her mother pretty well but her father was more resistant to manipulative tactics. In the end, the buck stopped with daddy, literally. When I told her good luck as she was leaving, she thanked me profusely. I wondered what I had done.

Linda Minor was discharged one day later, although I hardly noticed she was gone. I had almost nothing to do with her care once she told Artrell about her attraction to me. She was here almost two weeks and I'm not sure that we managed to do much for her, either. The only way we'll know (and I'll never find this information out) is if she is hauled back by the police into the Psychiatric Emergency Services, or "PES" as it's known. That would happen if she stops taking her medications. The one reason we have for hope is that the court has laid down the line that she cannot see her daughter unless she stays compliant with her medications and sees her court-appointed social worker. Given that her daughter seems to be the most important thing in her life, there's a possibility that she'll manage to overcome the paranoia and stay on the medication. *Then* the medication has to work, which isn't a certainty.

In the meantime, I picked up two new patients, both diagnosed with paranoid schizophrenia. My final week on 8 East might as well have been spent dealing with tiger sharks, so fearsome were these two women, who quickly found allies in one another and proceeded to terrorize the entire ward. My first introduction to Holly Eve, a 50 year-old African-American woman, was approaching her in the stimulation reduction room. She was singing Michael Jackson's "Billie Jean" very loudly, but at least keeping the tune. I came into the seclusion area and asked if I could talk to her. "Shut up, you motherfucking white devil," she said. Then she began to sing to Jesus, and she got down on her knees and delicately picked up her cup of orange juice.

"Well, if you don't want to talk to me, could you at least switch back to singing Billie Jean?" I asked. She slowly stood up, and I thought *there's something strange about the way she's holding that cup,* until I realized with about a second to spare that she's holding it like a projectile and means to douse me with the juice. When I stepped back, she started laughing, cackling actually.

"C'mon, baby, why don't you come over here and let me give you some orange juice?" she said. Then she got back down and started singing again. The next time I saw her several hours later, she had calmed down sufficiently to be released from seclusion, and she wrapped a sheet around her head in the manner of a turban and placed a dot of cold cream just between her eyebrows. She was calm enough to tell me that she wanted to talk to her daughter, and the mere mention of her daughter's name was enough to cause her to weep uncontrollably. She had come to the University Hospital the night before because she had threatened her daughter's fiancée, telling him that she was going to take a knife and cut him into little pieces. Since she had been released the month before from Marysville prison on a one-year sentence for assault, the future son-in-law took Holly at her word, and called the police.

Ms. Eve's partner in crime was, surprisingly, a 33 year-old white woman who had become just a *bit* too menacing to other residents in a group home. Kathy Baker has been circulating in and out of group homes for years, and appears to have exhausted the goodwill of the staff in most of the group homes in Hamilton and Butler counties. Holly just behaves weirdly, but one look at Kathy and you know she's mad. And she behaved that way as soon as she got to the ward. "Look, you motherfucker, I just want you to get *out* of my room and stay the *fuck* away from me as long as I'm here," were her first words to me when I asked her if we could talk. It didn't faze me much, though: She had said the same thing to every single staff person who had approached her.

The majority of patients in psych units do not like taking their medications. Sometimes they don't take it because they are paranoid about what's in the drugs, sometimes they don't take them because they don't want to admit that they are dependent on the drugs, and sometimes they don't take them because these drugs often have very unpleasant side effects. Holly, for instance, was refusing medications from the moment she arrived, and her refusal was probably rooted in all three reasons above. With Kathy, the problem wasn't compliance — she was perfectly willing to take medications. The problem was that the main medication that she was taking was haldol, one of the original antipsychotics used to treat schizophrenics and still a mainstay of treatment. But taking haldol regularly can lead to some unsightly side effects known collectively as *tardive dyskinesia*, which looks like the users have lost control over their bodies, writhing their limbs in a chaotic fashion. Kathy has tardive dyskinesia, and she could not be persuaded to change over to another antipsychotic with a lower side effect profile. Then again, she couldn't be persuaded to stop screaming *fuck you, assholes* at the staff—why should I be surprised that she wasn't going to try to switch her meds?

"Just give me my haldol, my ativan, and my cogentin, that's what I want," was the party line, and to her credit, she didn't deviate from it, unlike many patients, who change their tunes as to what drugs they'll take and what drugs they won't. For Kathy, who has bounced in and out of hospitals, and run a gauntlet of docs and meds, knowing that there are three drugs which work for her probably provides enough security that she isn't interested in trying anything new. But in the five or six days that I've seen her, twenty milligrams daily of haldol—which is a lot—haven't slowed her down a bit, and tardive dyskinesia is a permanent side effect.

Meds or no, Holly and Kathy have teamed up to create mass chaos on the hallway. They will start screaming or singing (Kathy's own contribution came one morning when she was pacing up and down the hallway singing "Ring My Bell"), get the other patients agitated, and a fight will ensue. Then, forget about it.

Wednesday, October 18

I worked the two shifts at Psych Emergency Services on Saturday night and Monday night. PES is a clearinghouse for most of the crisis psychiatric cases in the city. Here's how it works: You're John "Psycho Bob" Doe, and you've had a chronic illness with severe manic depression for years. You decided—after having a running conversation with God lasting approximately twenty straight hours without any need for sleep—that it's a good idea to go down to Fountain Square downtown and try to explain to passersby that you know how to bring peace and harmony to the world. You ask them if they are interested in seeing your private areas. Soon, an officer of the Cincinnati Police Department decides that you've had about enough.

From there, you can get whisked off to jail, where, if anyone is astute enough to recognize your behavior as being quite unusual instead of merely criminal, you might be evaluated by a court-appointed psychiatrist who will send you to the Pauline Warfield Lewis Center, a psychiatric hospital for criminals. You might fly under the radar screen and simply have a criminal trial. However, in this imaginary case your behavior is pretty clearly whacko, so the police will whisk you off to PES. From there, you can be held up to 72 hours against your will, at which point the psychiatrists may evaluate you and judge you unfit to be released. If that happens, they can request a probate hearing, and a magistrate over at the Lewis Center will hear the case and make a decision as to whether or not the person is fit to be released. (Missy Salina was one such patient.)

That's one kind of patient we see at PES. Another type is the chronic substance abuser who comes in to try to get clean. Typically, when these patients check themselves in they're doing it voluntarily, but as they go into withdrawal (sometimes before your very eyes) they decide it's not such a good idea and instead opt to go back out on the streets and score. That's not a problem if their number hasn't been called and they're still in the waiting room, but it is if they're already being evaluated, they've entered into the PES suite proper, which is a lockdown like the wards on the 8th floor, at which point they can't leave. They're stuck for the next 72 hours. And they don't like it. These patients will often end up in four-point restraints with several milligrams of a sedative drug called *ativan* in them. Ativan is pretty strong — my manic patient William a few weeks ago had to take more than a dozen milligrams of ativan before he got slowed down. It would only take a few to completely zonk a "normal" person.

I actually saw an alcoholic patient at PES who experienced this. While I was talking with the resident and social worker in the office, we heard screaming and hollering coming from the waiting room. The social worker and I bolted for the door, and we came out to see a guy shouting to be let in because he wanted to see a *fucking doctor, now! Goddamnit!* ("Fuck," if you haven't yet noticed, is an indispensable word when describing life on the psychiatric units.) Many of the people in the waiting room were perfectly healthy, non-psychiatric people who had escorted a family member there, and they were white with fear. Even the black people.

Once we opened the door for him, he decided that he didn't want to come in. So we had to negotiate with him. There were about three or four touch-and-go minutes, when it looked like he might try to beat the shit out of anyone who looked at him funny, but we managed to get him to come back. Whoosh! Four-point restraints and ativan almost immediately, because once he got in he decided it was time to get back out, and when he learned he couldn't he decided to throw a tantrum. When a severely drunk chronic alcoholic throws a tantrum, people can get their arms broken.

Two things about this encounter stick out in my mind, and both relate to the portrayal of drunk people on television. A TV drunk is always shown as stumbling around, slurring his or her every word, and when others approach the drunk, they always make gestures with their noses indicating that their breath reeks of alcohol. I've been drunk on many occasions in my adult life and I've been sober around drunk people many more times, and my observation is that it takes an heroic (or suicidal) amount of drinking to make a person stagger around and slur their words to the point of incomprehension. Not that you can't look and sound a little silly when you're drunk, but it's always exaggerated on television. And sure, people can smell alcohol on a drunk person's breath, but it takes a *lot* to be able to smell alcohol from, say, three feet away. This guy at PES would have been perfect for television. I smelled his breath as soon as I opened the door to the waiting room, and I was five feet away from him.

As I said, PES is designed to be a clearing house for *all* the psychiatric beds in the city. The patient enters the PES, and he or she is brought into an interview room by a social worker. The social worker will then interview the patient for as long as necessary to get a complete sense of what is going on, and they will in turn present the case to the doctor, who will also evaluate the patient. At that point, three things can happen. One is that the psychiatrist and social worker decide that the patient should be admitted to an inpatient unit. Once that decision is made, social workers get on the phone to find a bed somewhere in the city.

There aren't that many hospital psych wards in the area: Christ has one, as does the Good Samaritan, Mercy Franciscan, the VA, and of course the University has three wards. But the social worker has to call to see if there are beds available, if there are beds available for the right sex (many will have, say, *one* bed for a *woman* or *two* beds for *men*), and if the hospital will admit patients with such-and-such an insurance plan. Many of the private hospitals such as Christ aren't willing to eat the expense of treating a patient who has an insurance policy that doesn't cover inpatient psych (obviously those without insurance of any kind are out of the question), and those patients become slotted to go upstairs to the University wards, which takes on all comers.

Because many of the patients coming into PES are indigent, and because many of the hospitals with psych wards won't take indigent patients, University frequently gets backed up, which leads us to Option Number Two, which is that the patient is essentially put in deep-freeze down in PES until a bed opens up. When things get busy, that can mean up to a 48-hour stay in PES before they've even *begun* to get attention that even remotely earns the moniker of "therapeutic." Since PES is designed to treat emergent cases only, once a patient has been slotted for a bed, there's nothing that the nurses, physicians, or social workers can do for them. So they spend up to two, maybe even *three* days in a room about the size of a large classroom with dozens of other patients, locked up, getting very little attention.

The third option is that the team decides the patient is safe enough to leave the PES without being admitted to an inpatient unit. Patients who end up being shown the door to freedom are actually the *most* carefully scrutinized. Very little work is put into patients who are going to be admitted, because the inpatient treatment team is going to do a thorough evaluation of the patient once they arrive on the unit. But those that get released are treated with great skepticism, and it's because every doctor, nurse, and social worker (but especially every doctor) is paranoid about getting sued.

On Saturday night I interviewed a woman who was very depressed. She had made several attempts at taking her life, and had come in seeking help for her suicidal tendencies, but when we suggested that she was going to need to be admitted to the hospital for an inpatient stay since she was suicidal (a person who talks about wanting to commit suicide essentially instantly earns an automatic pass to inpatient status), she became deeply agitated with us. "Can't you see, if I don't show up for work this weekend, they're going to fire me and I'm not going to be able to pay my mortgage, and then what am I going to do for my son?" Well, I thought, that isn't the sound of a woman who's thinking about suicide. Even though she said that she couldn't remember ever having a happy day in the past twenty years, she still wanted to work at her job so that she could provide for her son. And since she had come to PES of her own accord, forcing her to go into a brief hospitalization against her will seemed to defeat the purpose in this case.

We did discharge her, but the conversation between the resident, the social worker, the nurse, and me about whether or not to admit her lasted for the better part of an hour. That was *after* she had received two hour-long evaluations. She left with some medications, probably equally as miserable as when she came in. I doubt very much that it did her any long-term good.

Thursday, October 19

The jail is where my "outpatient" rotation is. Since many psychiatrists don't work in the acute, inpatient settings that I've described over the past several pages, but rather work in offices usually seeing relatively functional patients, our clerkship includes an outpatient component once a week throughout our time in psych. Most of the options we had for the outpatient portion were at doctor's offices, and the patients were mostly garden-variety depressives, anxiety-sufferers, and hyperactive children.

I was fortunate enough to avoid this fate, and instead I was assigned to work in the Court Clinic down at the county jail. The jail is located at the northern tip of downtown, and is about a mile away from my home. The building is what you'd expect a jail to be: Forbidding, ugly, utilitarian. And that's the view from the *outside*. Inside it's worse. Concrete abounds except on the main floor, which is where the courtrooms are located, and even then the industrial-strength white granite-tiling is placed with such bureaucratic finesse that you wonder if we really *did* beat the Soviets in the Cold War.

Bouncing between the jail and her office in a much nicer county building across the street is my "preceptor," Dr. Jean Ottlinger. Preceptor isn't really the right word for her, since I'm not presenting patients to her and listening to her feedback. Instead, she's more like my guide. Each week is a show & tell of the criminal justice system; all I do is observe.

Ottlinger's job is, at its simplest, to evaluate whether or not certain inmates who have been incarcerated are fit to stand trial, or are "mentally competent." Mental competence does *not* mean the same thing as mental health. Jails are a psych med student's *dream* — if you spend long enough talking to the inmates, almost all of them will admit to or display some kind of psychopathology. Ottlinger isn't there to be a "therapeutic" psychiatrist and try to help a prisoner cope with his or her (usually his) mental problems. She's there to find out if they understood what they were doing was against the law, and did they understand that their violation had consequences.

Obviously not everybody gets a shot at the shrink. If prisoners were allowed this there would be an army of psychiatrists, psychologists, and social workers hired to keep up with the demand. Those inmates that receive a competency assessment have been pretty carefully screened by the attorneys and judges involved in the case. Even if they get assessed, they have very little chance of being deemed incompetent: About one percent of the accused are deemed unfit to stand trial. That's not to say that some of these criminals couldn't use psychiatric help, but the law is written to minimize the number of inmates judged incompetent to stand trial.

A good example of a guy who couldn't fit the bill was a 27 year-old black male who was in jail for burglary awaiting his trial. Dr. Ottlinger had assigned me to tag along with one of the social workers evaluating this gentleman. As we were walking over to the jail I looked at his chart. He had been in prison for one year for assault. Less than four weeks after his release he had been arrested for trying to steal some electronic equipment. He was stealing to make money to stay high, as he had been on a crack binge almost since the moment he was released from prison, the records indicated. "Hey, what's with this?" I asked. "I don't see any mental illness going on here besides drug addiction. That can't be enough, can it?"

"No, it can't," the social worker said. "I'm not sure how he got a referral, but he may have fired his old lawyer who had refused to ask for a referral, and somehow managed to convince his new lawyer that he needed an evaluation. We'll see."

We interviewed him in a small holding area between the inmates' living quarters and the main hallway on the fourth floor. I was struck by the guy's likeability. He told a pretty depressing story — depressing in that he was bouncing in and out of jail not for being particularly violent or malevolent, but for being addicted to drugs and trying to generate income to keep his habit going. After one stint in prison several years ago, he had managed for a two-year spell to stay clean, going to AA meetings, working the 12 steps, and regularly attending church. But eventually he got stressed out by life, and he went back to the crack. Now he is in for his third or fourth major offense, and this time he isn't going to get a year when he gets convicted — and he will be convicted. This time he will probably get five to ten. That's if he's declared competent, which he is.

I was also struck by his "psychiatric history." Though he didn't know it, he was a classic case of depression, and based on what he said, the depression started prior to the crack use.

It's quite possible that the crack was a form of self-medication, since about half of all patients with major depression also abuse drugs or alcohol. His relapses aren't that surprising, since many addicts must quit more than once until they manage to quit for good.

But some of the people Dr. Ottlinger interviews are truly *nuts*. Once when I accompanied the doctor we had a bonanza morning, where two out of two people we interviewed were declared incompetent and were probated to the Lewis Center. They both had chronic schizophrenic-type diseases. One had gotten picked up at Fountain Square for exposing his penis to passersby, eventually making the mistake of flashing a female cop. His file was filled with minor arrests for such behavior, multiple hospitalizations in state institutions, and various diagnoses of mental illness.

The other guy was arrested for reasons that we weren't able to figure out based on what "Willie," the prisoner, had told us. He was the heir to a family fortune, but had been diagnosed with schizophrenia for nearly thirty years. It wasn't hard to tell that he was in bad shape. He was wearing a pair of glasses, but missing one lens, which seemed not to bother him in the slightest. The side with the lens was virtually pressed up against his eyeball. When we asked him why he had gotten arrested, he began a five-minute monologue that, try as we may, we couldn't hope to understand.

"Look, I needed to go get my check," he said toward the end, leaning over the table to talk to us confidentially, his breath indescribably foul. Try as he might, there wasn't going to be any privacy in this room, where inmates and staff were shuffling back and forth on their way to various sites of administrative processing. "It was about two in the morning, and it was raining. I like to go out walking when it's raining, because I can think more clearly."

"You were going to pick up your check at two in the morning? Who's your payee?" Dr. Ottlinger asked, referring to the Social Security Disability Income checks that many non-institutionalized mentally ill patients receive. Part of the requirement is that such people have a "payee," someone who can distribute the checks each month and make sure they are compliant with their medications. Obviously it wasn't standard operating procedure to drop by one's payee at 2 a.m.

"Christ Hospital. I went out walking toward Christ..."

"Wait. Where were you when you left for Christ?"

"Walnut Hills." That's about an hour's walk away.

"Why didn't you just wait until morning?"

That stumped him. "Look, the police came and picked me up, and then here I ended up. And look, I want you to take a look at my dentures." He pulled out his lower dentures, which had a green covering toward the back that appeared to be mold. Dr. Ottlinger abruptly got up and nearly pushed me out of the way.

"That's it. Thanks very much for your time," Dr. Ottlinger said.

Willie was deemed incompetent with Dr. Ottlinger's input that very afternoon.

Friday, October 20   Children's Hospital Psych Ward

Nellie Woodstock, by all rights, shouldn't be in Children's Hospital at all. She appears unusually bright for a nine year-old, and has multiple talents: Good at drawing and math, verbally sophisticated, analytical. She has a very nasty temper, though, and while hitting your parents is one matter, hitting your younger siblings is another matter entirely. And hitting your teacher? Well, that earns you a ticket to the psych ward.

Her official diagnosis is "oppositional defiant disorder" which is a relative of the diagnosis "conduct disorder," both of which used to be diagnosed as "problem child," or, in more subdued language, "difficult." Nellie has temper tantrums, and can't be easily controlled by her single mother. Her father, divorced from mom for the last two years, told me over the phone that he's never had any problems with her, didn't understand what all the fuss was about, and thought that mom needed to recognize her own inflexibility towards her, because that, as he saw it, was the major problem.

I spoke with him over the phone for about a half-hour

yesterday, and later that morning mom called. She was revved up, quite clearly angry about the situation with Nellie, the disruption that it was causing to her life and her other children, and believed that part of the problem lay in her former husband's coddling of her. After setting up a meeting with my resident and attending, I called them back to arrange a family meeting, with the hopes that a cease-fire could be induced for the welfare of Nellie.

After I got off with both of them, I knew that it was a messy divorce, and that children caught in the crossfire of such divorces become casualties, and unless we got them to snap out of their mutual hatred we weren't going to get anywhere. I also understood that there was only very rarely one party to blame for such family problems, that the truth of who was responsible was a sticky matter at best to sort out. That said, my own feelings were that I liked the father, who seemed reasonable and pleasant, and I didn't like the mother, who seemed edgy and bitter. I knew that my taking sides wasn't of any use to anyone, but I had to be aware of my gut reaction before I could check it at the door.

We managed to convene a meeting for this morning, and oh, what a difference it makes to see the family in action. Mom *was* edgy and bitter, but by the end of the meeting I was more than halfway in understanding her edginess and bitterness. Dad was, essentially, a marshmallow—according to mom, he didn't try to behave like Nellie's father, he behaved like her best friend. He imposed no discipline on her, didn't try to establish rules or expectations. Some of this is obviously subjective, but the single fact that changed my view was when I discovered that when she stays with him in his apartment, the two *sleep together in the same bed*. How's *that* for sending mixed messages?

Still, as sympathetic as I became toward the mother and as unsympathetic as I became toward the father, I knew that wasn't any more helpful, and although the attending and resident were in the room, I decided, after listening to several minutes of accusation and counter-accusation, that I was going to step up to the plate. "Listen," I said as gingerly as possible,

117

"I think one thing that we need to do here is remember that we're here because Nellie is in a good deal of trouble, and she needs our help. I'm sure you'll both agree that she's a very talented girl, and that the more she sees divisiveness between you, the more stressed she'll become, and she's acting out that stress. So although you have differences with one another, I think that Nellie will benefit if you, collectively, don't send contradictory signals. It seems to me that your goal today, above all else, is to come walking out of this room as a united front. You've *got* to support each other's decisions—even when you don't like them—when dealing with her. What do you think?"

I got mostly blank stares, like I had just asked a Palestinian and an Israeli to agree on the occupation of Jerusalem.

"Mr. Woodstock," I said. "You're with her mostly on the weekends, is that right? Well, I think one thing you need to agree to is to keep the same studying rules that apply when she's at home during the week. Will you be able to enforce those rules? *Her* rules?" I said, pointing to Mrs. Woodstock.

He nodded glumly.

"Mrs. Woodstock," I said. "Will you avoid criticizing Mr. Woodstock in front of Nellie when she returns from the weekends? Will you respect the rules that he's set for Nellie if her schoolwork is done when she's with him according to your rules?"

She looked me over. "Yes, I will."

"So we have an agreement to walk out of here today, out of this meeting, as a united front?" I finished.

"Yes, I agree," she said.

"Yes, I agree," he said.

"But he's *got* to get some counseling, or we're not going to make any headway," she quickly added.

"Me? You've got to stop being the control freak that you love to be," he responded.

"I can't believe you," she replied.

This wasn't quite what I had in mind when I used the word "agreement."

Saturday, October 28

There are two attendings that run the inpatient Child Psych department, both of whom were away the better part of the last week due to a conference they both attended. One is Patricia Cartwell, who is new to the unit, and has been there something like a few months. She looks like my third-grade teacher — or anyone's third-grade teacher, for that matter. She's unattractive in a gender-neutral kind of way, the kind of woman who doesn't much remind you of the concept "woman" at all. Unfair, you say? Yes, that's right. But, dammit, this is psychiatry after all, and I might as well be honest about my gut reactions in this chapter.

Cartwell as a shrink is equally unimpressive to me. She was Nellie Woodstock's doctor, and when Nellie met her last Wednesday, she reacted to Cartwell as she did to any authority figure: She got pissy the minute she heard something that she didn't like. In this case, she didn't like being told she had to talk to Dr. Cartwell about why she was here.

"I don't want to talk to you," she said matter-of-factly to Cartwell.

"But you *have* to talk to me," Cartwell replied, not especially sweetly.

I was so stunned by that reply that I thought I misunderstood what was going on. Telling a kid who has issues with authority that she *has* to do something is only going to make her say that she *won't* do it, right? I'm no pro, but it seemed like exactly the opposite tactic you'd want to take.

"Well, I'm not *going* to talk to you," Nellie replied, more testily now.

"*Oh* yes you are!" Cartwell retorted, becoming more animated. As I said, at first I couldn't believe it, but it was becoming clear to me that Cartwell was getting into exactly the kind of fight that Nellie wanted to have. She was getting wrapped up in Nellie's game. I sat watching the whole conversation escalate into a fight; it felt like I was watching a car accident, like it was awful to look at but I could do nothing to stop it.

"You know what, *fuck you*," Nellie said.

"You're not going to use that kind of language around here, young lady!" Cartwell said. "And if you're not going to talk to me, you're going to lose all of your privileges, and you'll have to stay here in your room! Is that what you want?" Nellie just sat and glared. "Well then, fine!" Dr. Cartwell said and stormed out of the room. On her way out the door, she added, "You'll come to me when you're ready to talk, and then we'll *discuss* giving you some privileges back!"

This is a *child* psychiatrist? Gracious.

I sat in the room with Nellie for several minutes on the opposite bed, not saying anything. Then I pulled up a chair to her bed, looked at her, and said, "Nellie, what was that all about?"

Tears now were starting to come down the corners of her eyes. "I just don't want to talk to her," she said, fighting the tears.

"Nellie, listen, you're having a tough enough day as it is. I don't want to see you try to fight everyone around you, especially the people who are trying to help you out. You sure you don't want to talk to me, or Dr. Cartwell, or someone else on the staff? We're all trying to make this thing better so you can get out of here."

"I want you to leave," she said to me.

"Okay," I said. "I'll leave. If you want to talk, you know where to find us. I hope that you come to us soon, because I know we can help." I left to go to class not long after this, and found out Thursday morning that later in the afternoon Nellie agreed to talk to Dr. D'Alessio, the child psych fellow, but *not* to Dr. Cartwell.

That Thursday I grabbed my classmate Bryant and asked him what he thought of Cartwell. "She seems okay to me," he said. "You know, her specialty is in autistic children." Children without much emotion, without rage, who don't try to manipulate people, I thought. *Now* it makes more sense. She's a bit autistic herself.

Incidentally, Nellie was released earlier in the week, and what good it did I'll likely never know. My sense is that without intensive family therapy she'll be just as pissed ten years from now, if not more, as she is currently. Under normal circumstances, I'd think that she will turn into one of life's casualties, given the pathologic nature of her family's relations. But she has one thing going for her that none of the other kids I've seen so far on the ward possess: Stunning intelligence. Whether that will provide enough lift for her to extricate herself from the mess that is her mother and father remains to be seen, but that magnificent talent locked inside her cranium might help her figure the way out.

Did our little hospitality-and-crisis-psychotherapy help her? Not much, is my guess.

Ψ Ψ Ψ Ψ Ψ Ψ Ψ Ψ Ψ

The other attending psychiatrist is Bob Tomlinson, the unofficial guru of the floor. Tomlinson — "Doctor Bob" — is charismatic, friendly, and able to interact with children on their level. Which isn't to say that he himself is a child. It's just that he manages to accomplish an extremely hard task — to get the kids to talk to him, not like he's a "doctor," but like someone that they *trust*. And part of getting the kids to trust him involves being a little silly and playful.

Take, for instance, "music therapy." Music therapy is Doctor Bob's version of the kind of sing-along that Barney-the-Purple-Dinosaur does on TV. He plays guitar, and sings out various songs, playing games through the singing. The games are intended to get them to recognize the importance of working cooperatively, being nice to others, learning self-discipline, that kind of thing — he'll strum really quickly and have everyone run around the room, but when he stops, the children have to return to a seat and cannot move until he starts playing again. With each successive silence, he waits longer and longer. The kids see it as sheer fun, but the longer they manage to sit, the more they learn to be patient and control their impulses.

Though I mention that hack Barney, Tomlinson's music is much more like the Looney Tunes from a generation ago, where his songs will be laced with pop-culture references way above the kids' heads. I've heard bits and pieces of the Beatles, the Eagles, the Who, Jimi Hendrix, and Neil Young run through his musical games. The kids aren't thinking about all that heavy stuff that they have to deal with in "real" therapy, when they're in a room talking to an adult about being beaten, or raped, or molested by some family member. They're just kids having fun. Tomlinson's got them learning while they do that, and for many of them it's the most important part of the day.

Tomlinson's pretty well-known among the medical students. He spends a fair amount of time talking with the medical students, which is difficult for a busy attending. He is also willing to discuss topics with the students that ostensibly have no bearing on medical school whatsoever, like what makes us scared, what we hate, what we want to do with ourselves in life. My classmate Andathi is pretty uncomfortable with this part of his shtick. "Dag, man, like, I don't need to have him sit there and psychoanalyze me, you know? Everything I say, that cat wants to know what it *really means*," he said in exasperation after the second or third day.

I really don't know what to make of Andathi. He's definitely a likeable guy, pretty easygoing. But that "cat," Dr. Tomlinson—everyone is a "cat" in Andathi-speak—gets way under his skin. He's deeply uncomfortable with the kind of introspection that Tomlinson encourages him to do, and that discomfort makes *me* uncomfortable about *him*.

One day we had followed Tomlinson to his outpatient rounds with two other students who were assigned to his outpatient section. At the end of the afternoon the five of us were kicking around various topics, mostly psychopharm questions that we had about this drug's side effects or that drug's indications for use in children. Tomlinson got off on a tangent; he started talking about when non-psychiatric doctors don't understand the psychological motivations that both they and their patients have, then they often *contribute* to their patients' problems by getting angry with them.

"Well, *I* don't get angry," Andathi said offhandedly.

Tomlinson glanced at him. "You don't?"

"No, I never get angry."

"Steven, do you believe him?"

"No, I don't."

"Andathi, Steven doesn't believe you. Why is that?"

"I don't know, but I don't get angry."

"Never?"

"No."

"Do you have an omentum?" Tomlinson asked. An 'omentum' being a part of the gut.

"What?"

"Do you have an omentum?"

"Yeah, sure I do."

"Well, do you have a limbic system?"

"What?"

"Do you have a limbic system? Because if you're brain is hard-wired like most everyone else's, then you have a limbic system, and that limbic system produces very powerful, primitive feelings like anger. If you're not aware that you get angry, man, can bad things happen."

So the conversation went.

Monday, October 30

The last patient that I'll be taking care of before I finish psychiatry is Bernie, who I picked up Thursday morning. Bernie is a ten year-old black child. He is *enormous* relative to his peers. No one on the wards is even close to his size, which by my reckoning is eighty or ninety pounds. To me, he's a kid, but to his peers, he must be Mean Joe Green.

Bernie is a sweet kid. Really. He likes other kids, he likes the staff, he likes playtime and the activities that they've set up for him here at the hospital. In some ways, my guess is that Bernie would love to *stay* in the hospital, with its structure, its warmth, and its safety. This is exactly the opposite way that Nellie, a white, bright suburban kid, viewed her experience: Her environment possesses those qualities already.

Why is this sweet kid in the hospital? Because—sit down for this—he drove a pencil through another child's hand while on the bus ride home from school. The other child apparently called him "fat," and he reached for his pencil, grabbed the child's hand, and in one swift downward stroke, landed the pencil directly through its middle. When I first met him the only thing I knew was that his psych diagnosis was "intermittent explosive disorder," and after meeting this happy child I wondered what was going on with him. Then I read the specifics of the history and I thought that intermittent explosive disorder was an understatement.

This was not the first time Bernie has had a violent outburst; even though only a second grader, he's already been suspended several times for fighting with other children and for striking out at teachers. This most recent incident was simply the worst. He will be expelled from the school, and somehow the Cincinnati City Schools must try to figure out where to place this walking time bomb.

Bernie's family life is more representative of the kind of life lived by most of the children who end up here. Nellie was an unusual kid for being suburban and from a family of relative wealth; Bernie's "family" — which consists of a haggard mother caring for two other children and a father halfway through a three-year stint in prison for beating mother to a pulp — lives in the tough, drug-ridden neighborhood of Over-The-Rhine. It's very likely that Bernie witnessed horrible acts of violence between his father and mother on a daily basis for years, may have been a victim himself (though his mother insists to the contrary) and his own violence is only an imitation of what he's seen at home.

His mom doesn't work, so there isn't going to be any insurance company lining up to foot the ten thousand dollar bill that Bernie was going to run up in a one-week stay; that meant that the hospital was going to eat the expense of housing him, which in turn meant that there was going to be a bean counter from somewhere in the bowels of the hospital who would be chomping at the bit to get this kid out the door.

What we're going to do for Bernie is precious little. The child psych unit is meant to be used strictly for emergent stabilization, meaning once the staff gets them out of the danger zone (whether a danger to themselves or others), they are sent home and outpatient follow-up is arranged. Bernie will benefit from the so-called "token economy" that we provide, which allows kids to earn tokens for good behavior that they can turn in for various rewards—free time, special time with a staff person and whatnot—and he'll certainly profit from the enormous volume of attention foisted upon him.

But ten days here—the maximum someone's going to agree to keep Bernie (it's more likely to be five)—can't even begin to address the demons wrapping themselves around this boy. Even a third-year can plainly see that he needs to be in intensive behavioral therapy and psychotherapy for a long time if he's going to have a shot at turning out to be a decent kid. The kind of money that it would cost to provide these programs is way beyond what anyone is willing to pay at the front end. He will have some follow-up arranged, though, even if it is a mere pittance of what he requires. But even that won't be of much use, because after a few days of dealing with his mother, who's been bruised and battered by life in ways simply unimaginable to me, it's become clear to me that he'll never make it to any follow-up appointments. To expect her to have a calendar and plan and keep a meeting weeks or months in advance is expecting way too much.

I said that the cost to provide adequate help to Bernie is beyond what anyone wants to pay "on the front end." I say that because, after several conversations with Dr. Tomlinson and the nursing staff, there's pretty much a consensus that we'll be paying even greater expenses on the *back* end. This will occur when grown-up Bernie, no better able to control his anger, will beat the shit out of his girlfriend, or, instead of driving a pencil through another's hand, will send a bullet through another's head. Then we'll be paying $30,000 a year to house him in a jail.

Tuesday, October 31

Today was another tête-à-tête between Andathi and Dr. Tomlinson. Following the afternoon child psych clinic, Andathi and I were sitting around shooting the breeze while Dr. Tomlinson finished up with a last patient. The subject had turned to grades and class standing. We were also swapping various rumors about the board scores of some classmates—those that were ridiculously high, or those that were ridiculously low. While exchanging what we knew about this or that person, many of whom were our friends, Andathi spoke about a few classmates who didn't much impress me. They did have impressive board scores, which was how their names came up; their manner with patients, or even other classmates, I found less impressive.

"Man, those cats are so *smart*," he said. "They're the most intelligent people in the school."

I tried to bite my tongue. None of them struck me as more intelligent than the average student, they simply had high board scores because they spent more hours in the library. Before I began to reply, a voice suddenly came from behind us, saying, "Tell me, Andathi, what defines intelligence?" We wheeled around to see Dr. Tomlinson, already finished seeing his patient, smiling down on us, waiting to hear his response.

"What do you mean?" asked Andathi.

"Well, you say these guys are smart. What quality is it that makes you regard these classmates as being special?"

"They all got above two forty-five on their boards."

"And that's what makes them intelligent?"

"Well, it's a sign, that's for sure."

"Do you know what your IQ is, Andathi?"

"What?"

"Have you ever wondered what your IQ is? Do you wonder how people measure intelligence?"

"Not really. I have no idea what my IQ is."

"Steven, do you know what your IQ is?"

"What's the standard deviation?" I asked.

"Say it's fifteen with a mean of one hundred."

"Then my guess is it's about one fifteen."

"Why is that your guess?"

"I don't know, really. I know that I'm smart, but I also know that I'm not *really* smart."

"Interesting. What do you think the smartest doctors do?"

"They get the best jobs, don't you think?" Andathi asked.

"It depends on what you mean. Based on my experience, there are three kinds of doctors. The smartest ones go into research. Average doctors make good clinicians and spend their careers taking care of their patients pretty well." He paused.

"And the third group?" I asked.

"The least intelligent doctors usually end up making the most money," he said with a wink.

Friday, November 3

I am—mercy—finished with the psych rotation. It ended with a thud. The exam was astonishingly difficult. It was a two-hour, 100-question national, standardized exam, better known as a "shelf" exam. My brain felt like mashed potatoes by the end. I never had considered that the psychiatry exam would have a much higher level of difficulty than the surgery exam.

I said goodbye to Dr. Tomlinson when we had a bonding session of sorts yesterday when we went out for lunch together. He pitched to me an idea about doing my residency in child psych while doing research in behavioral genetics, a subject that interests me. It's an idea that I'm at least going to try on. Tomlinson's a good guy to learn from, and having a real mentor that I know and like is something I've never really had in my adult life. Plus Children's Hospital is supposed to be the real deal—one of the top pediatric hospitals in the country, with lots and lots of money for research coming in and lots of good researchers doing work here. I don't think the child psych residency is as top-flight as the pediatric medicine department at Children's, but it's still a very good place to make connections.

I'll think about it but I'm pretty sure I'm not going to take him up on the offer. Mostly I'm flattered that someone tried to recruit me. The truth is that I just can't imagine myself doing child psychiatry. I also am skeptical of how much good we're actually doing the kids, not because we *can't* do them any good but because they just don't have enough time in the hospital. These kids are mostly coming from total chaos, where the mother's getting beaten by the boyfriend or husband, or she's a druggie, or a prostitute, or both, the patients themselves have been sexually molested or have witnessed it, et cetera. Seven-to-ten days in the psych ward with one or two medications thrown in is not going to reverse that kind of trauma.

Several of the staff have told me that the kids used to stay for a month or two. "We used to all be crying when they left," one of the women who has worked there for over ten years said to me. "We got to know those kids really well. They practically became family. Now there's so many of them, and they're coming through so quickly, that we hardly get to know any of them at all." The insurance companies are mostly responsible for this sea change. Kids who need potentially months of intensive training on how to cope with the insanity around them instead get about a week and are sent off with meds.

That's not the kind of profession I want to go into.

four

a six-week vacation,

otherwise known as "electives"

Sunday, November 5

The third year curriculum at University of Cincinnati is split into two halves: One half consists of "The Big Three" of pediatrics, internal medicine, and OB/GYN, while the other half consists of surgery, psychiatry, family medicine, and six weeks devoted to "electives." Since students must decide what field they wish to pursue early into the fourth year, UC allows students to explore smaller specialties in medicine during the third year with these electives should they want to apply to those programs.

Therefore, we can choose two two-week electives from the following list: ER, ophthalmology, neurology, dermatology, urology, neurosurgery, oncology, orthopedic surgery, physical medicine and rehabilitation, and otolaryngology (or ENT*). ER is the most sought-after elective—so popular, in fact, that many students who want to take the elective cannot due to its long waiting list. Of these, I chose oncology and neurology.

I'll cap it off with radiology. There isn't a medical field out there that isn't reliant to some degree on radiology, so the medical school requires it. The radiology elective has traditionally been a favorite among medical students since we're required to work very few hours, and the radiologists expect us only to breathe and maybe smile at their jokes once in a while. Thus it's been known at this institution for many years as "the radiation vacation."

Indeed, the elective period in general is acknowledged as the one period during the third year where one can take it easy. Getting a high-pass instead of an honors in urology isn't going to kill you (unless, of course, you want to match in urology), and so most of us view the elective time as a chance to kick back, relax, and enjoy the moment. In my case, since surgery and psych are behind me and the Big Three are looming around the corner, the electives couldn't have come at a better time.

So the following pages will be brief entries about my chosen electives. Since the school's intention during this period

---

* ENT stands for "Ear, Nose, Throat."

is to provide a bird's-eye view of these specialties rather than cultivate clinical skills in any meaningful way, I'm certain that my education will be much more hands-off. I also suspect that I won't be spending the same intensive time with my *real* teachers, the patients, as I have previously. I learn my best when I'm responsible for others, but I won't object to a few weeks on easy street.

Neurology

Monday, November 6

The guy who I'm going to be working with mostly on this rotation is Chad Kantor, a youngish guy new to the faculty who did his residency in Neurology at the University of Michigan. *I* look older than him. From what I've seen of him so far I may well *feel* older than him, as he's mentioned his love of the TV show *South Park* about oh, say, five or six times today. He's very enthusiastic about what he does, though, and even though I have no real desire to go into neurology I appreciate his cheerleading.

It's pretty clear based on how things went today that this is a very loose course in terms of what you're required to do. They gave me a schedule with two or three things I can attend, simultaneously, on each day. Kantor said that I should try to get as many different experiences in as possible so that I can see "all the different things that neurologists get to do" and made it clear that nobody was going to be standing around going, "now where's that medical student?" I immediately translated this information into *wow! a few afternoons off!* Which is probably an indicator of just how much I want to do neurology.

It's also clear that the neuro faculty view these two weeks more as a chance to recruit potential residents and less as an opportunity to teach the medical students how to do a good neuro history and physical. I got a whiff of the recruitment pitch when William Bostwick, the department chairman, came up to me after a faculty meeting and introduced himself. That, in and of itself, seems a big deal — department chairs generally aren't in the habit of troubling themselves with medical students.

He didn't beat around the bush very long. "So, what are you thinking about for residency? I'm assuming that you're thinking about neurology since you've signed up for this elective," he said.

Hmmm. How to phrase this gracefully? "Oh, I *am* thinking about neurology," I started off. "When I signed up for these electives, I was thinking about both neuro and infectious diseases. I'm considering doing my residency in internal medicine and doing a fellowship in ID, but nothing's off the table at the moment. My mind's pretty open."

So I lied. I'm pretty set on going the medicine route, but what could I say? The department chair doesn't want to hear that the single third-year student who's doing the neuro rotation wants to go into something *else*; he wants to hear the story of a person who suddenly thinks—yes! Yes! *This* is what I want to do! And who am I to disabuse him of this view?

Incidentally, this maneuver is a favorite among the more cutthroat-minded students in our class. Suppose that you, student at the good-but-not-great Med School U., want to do surgery at Cornell. You sailed through your first two years in the basic science courses (which are based exclusively on standardized tests) at the top of the class. You spent your one free summer in medical school[*] working in the laboratory of a prominent surgeon who does research. You did extremely well on the boards. Now you've come to the third year. You've got pretty good social skills. You *should* do well, but what can you do to give you that edge above other students to keep you at the head of the class?

Simple. When you start OB/GYN, you let it slide into casual conversation with the residents and the faculty that there's nothing more in life that you would like to do than

---

[*] Most medical schools in the US allow only one free summer, the summer between the first and second years. After the second year ending in early May, students prepare for the boards, which they can take anywhere from late May to late June. The third year begins around July 1, and aside from the two weeks of vacation around Christmas, it runs straight into the fourth year, which continues through the summer and keeps on going. However, the fourth year has more opportunities for electives and vacations.

be an obstetrician. In fact, it's been your dream to be an obstetrician since the birth of your little sister when you were eight years old. You wax eloquent about being present at the beginning of one's life—*what a great honor it is to participate in the birth of children,* or something like that—and you ask attendings about good programs for residency. You never miss an opportunity to show how dedicated you are to this specialty. If no one suspects it's a ruse, at evaluation time you get a little bump in your grade because attendings are more likely to show a little favoritism to students who wants to go into their specialty.

Then, when you've finished your rotation and you've taken your test, you start Medicine, and lo! you realize that it's really *Medicine* that you've wanted to do all along. You say the same kinds of things to the Medicine attendings that you had said only weeks ago to the OB/GYN people. It's an effective way of doing business, even if technically the core clerkships aren't supposed to favor students who want to go into that specialty. Many of us students believe that, even if only subconsciously, an attending will inflate the grade of a student who expresses a desire to go into that field.

I've heard stories from the fourth-year class about their classmates doing this, but so far I haven't heard any rumors about one of my classmates pulling this stunt. My guess is that most students, when asked by an attending about their career plans, will answer in the way that I did to Bostwick: Haven't ruled anything out yet. That way you haven't outright lied, but you allow attendings to draw their own conclusions—conclusions that just might benefit your grade.

According to Kantor, Bostwick is a really big kahuna in the stroke community. "Steven, there aren't many programs here in Cincinnati that are internationally renowned," he told me after Bostwick introduced himself, "but our Stroke Team is one of them. And it's mostly because of Will Bostwick." He said this with as much gravitas as could be mustered from a man in his mid-thirties who doesn't look a day over 18.

Wednesday, November 8

On Wednesdays the neuro department does a teaching session for the medical students. It's mostly for the fourth-year students, since about a dozen of them are in the department, while there's only me from the third year. It is run by Dr. Jason Cuinan, one of the senior staff in the department. When you first catch a glimpse of him you might be moved to some form of pity. He has a neurological disorder (I don't know what it is and don't consider it my business to ask) that limits his ability to move his limbs, so he gets around in a little scooter.

If you did think that he was an object of pity, you'd be sorely mistaken. His presence is so dominating that hardly anyone notices the scooter after a time, and most of the students talk about him in reverent tones: How he did his training at the Mayo Clinic and is one of the smartest guys in the entire medical center, how he is among the finest clinical educators in the medical school, et cetera.

I don't know from the Mayo, but what I admire most about Cuinan is his impish sense of humor. During our second year, in pathology, he gave a lecture about various neurologic diseases. One of the diseases he discussed was *kuru*, a so-called 'prion' disease, not unlike Creutzfeld-Jakob disease that humans picked up from the "Mad Cow" epidemic a few years ago. Kuru is transmitted by the funereal practices of some Pacific Islanders, practices that include ritual cannibalism. Cuinan thought it proper to put in a note about this, and in our lecture notes he wrote, "Take home message from the South Pacific: *Do not eat your ancestors' brains as a ceremonial sign of respect.* Prions are weird — proteins capable of creating a 'destructive chain letter' in your brain. Prions are not destroyed by standard sterilization. Chlorox seems to do the job, but not an option for an infected patient."

When we came into the teaching session today, Cuinan looked around and said, "Now who's the third-year?"

I indicated I was present.

"Where's your case?"

"Um, what case?"

"Didn't you know you were supposed to present?"

"Actually, I thought I was supposed to present next week. I thought that's what my schedule said."

"Oh. Okay, we'll put you on the hot seat next week. Fair enough, I'll just take some cases out of my old file, then."

Just like that—no harassment, no lecture on responsibility, just a quick shrug and he moved on. I almost felt nostalgic for surgery. Cuinan went on to do a case discussion about a garden-variety migraine headache. After we moved through a discussion on the kinds of questions you would want to ask the patient when taking their medical history, what other kinds of diseases you might want to rule out, and what tests you would consider ordering, he led us into discussion about the treatment for migraine.

"So, what do you think of as your first-line med?" Cuinan asked us.

Someone called out the answer that we had all been trained to give: "Triptans." Triptans are a class of drugs, the most famous of which is sumatriptan, whose trade name is Imitrex.

"Right, triptans. Now, does anyone know how much sumatriptan costs?"

Someone with a Palm Pilot started poking around and eventually told us that ninety tablets of either 25 or 50 milligrams cost about $125. Palm Pilots are indispensable to medical students; a program named "Epocrates" contains a small textbook's worth of information you can carry in your pocket, even including the cost of the drug, which the fourth-year banged out in less than two seconds. Hardly any third-year is without a Palm Pilot for this reason.

Cuinan said, "Okay, now you've all been told that the triptans are the drug of choice for treating migraines. That's because people have been buying the stuff that those drug reps hand out in the free lunches that they give once a week. But what those flyers *aren't* telling you about is that the literature indicates they aren't much more effective than Tylenol in head-to-head trials. And how much does an over-the-counter medication cost? I don't know, a couple of bucks, maybe. It's certainly not one hundred twenty-five dollars."

"But then how can those drug companies make their claims about its effectiveness?" I asked.

"Because they're comparing their effectiveness to placebo, not to the other ways you can treat migraine," he said. "Look, if your patient looks at you funny when you tell them to use an over-the-counter, just look them in the eye, lean in confidentially and say, 'I recommend Excedrin *Migraine* for my patients.' It's not really different from regular Excedrin, but they'll feel better about using it."

Friday, November 10

Today's lesson was in how doctors administer serious pain to their patients. At the morning clinic I witnessed a procedure known as an "EMG." To medical types, it stands for "electromyelogram"; to patients, it stands for "torture."

An EMG is a test that allows neurologists to observe how well or poorly the body's electrical circuitry is working. For instance, an EMG can be used to document carpal tunnel syndrome: Patients with the syndrome cannot conduct electrical signals from the brain through the median nerve in the wrist the same way that normal, healthy people can. You can confirm a provisional diagnosis of carpal tunnel syndrome (as well as other neurologic disorders) by the EMG. You do an EMG by sticking needles in various places in the body (adjacent to whichever nerve you wish to study), sending an electrical pulse through the needle so as to transmit it to the nerve, and then looking for the conduction downstream of that nerve through another needle. An EMG is, quite literally, a series of tiny electrocutions visualized on a computer screen.

I saw three EMGs during the clinic session, and not one patient managed to complete the procedure without repeatedly yowling in pain. Since this was a residents' clinic, the EMGs were being performed by the residents themselves, with Dr. Cuinan behind them, quizzing them about the anatomy of the regions they were sticking, as well as the dermatomal distribution of the nerves they were trying to study (dermatomes are regions of the surface of the body that correspond to regions in the spinal cord where the neurons live). One of the residents, a Chinese grad with fairly halting English, was screwing up the answers on the first patient, and Cuinan was nonplussed.

"You know, I think you had better make sure you know the anatomy really well before you start sticking needles in people," Cuinan said, obviously pissed. I've never seen him like this before; his tone instantly reminded me of the senior surgeons chastising their residents. Only Cuinan seemed even more angry and dismissive. Meanwhile, the patient was sitting on the exam table, coping with two medium-sized needles in his arm, occasionally receiving shocks, *listening* to this conversation. It must not have been, pardon the pun, a real shot in the arm in terms of his confidence.

"I think you need to go back to the anatomy book before we let you go at this again," Cuinan said with disgust. "I think it's my turn to take over." He then moved up to the patient, apologized for the banter, and started chit-chatting with the patient to ease the tension. The procedure continued, causing no less pain for the patient, while Dr. Cuinan continued to ask the chastened resident about nerve distributions, dermatomes, and evidence of diagnostic signs on the monitor.

When doing general surgery, I saw interns and residents struggle to learn how to perform procedures correctly. They made mistakes, as apprentices do, but I didn't find it alarming since the patient was fast asleep and the mistakes themselves were harmless to the patient in the long run. While the mistakes of this resident were equally harmless, the patient was wide awake, fully aware that he was practice material. That has to be terrifying.

Wednesday, November 15

Today was "go out and see a private-practice neurologist" day, and I had the pleasure of driving *way* out to the far eastern suburbs to meet Vincent Cable, a product of the UC neurology residency and a guy apparently still well connected to the department, since he's willing to pick up medical students fairly regularly without much complaint. I can understand working with a medical student for a month, because in that time you can develop a relationship and actually have a meaningful impact on that student's education, but it must be somewhat annoying to have a parade of medical students coming through your office, each for only one afternoon. Yuck!

Fortunately, Doc Cable and I hit it off right from the start. Cable's clearly a special guy. Not only does he have the touch with patients, he thinks about his patients' needs in a manner totally different from anything that I've seen before. In addition to his nine-to-five, medication-prescribing, reflex-hammer-tapping, white-coat-wearing routine, he's incorporated other elements into his practice. A few afternoons a week he shares his office with a massage therapist, with whom he has a business arrangement, shuffling patients her way and sharing the rent with her. He also has a "music therapy" group that meets a few evenings throughout the month; the goal of the group is to use music as part of a relaxation program. Patients who want their doctor to think outside the box should go check out Cable.

I don't want to get into a long drawn-out discussion of so-called "alternative medicine," but in the meantime let me say this: I think most of what people call alternative medicine is sheer quackery, but likewise I think Vince Cable is the model for what MDs should be trying to do with their practices. I didn't need to spend three years in medical school to know that a massage *feels good*, and that regular relaxation contributes to an improved quality of life. Why shouldn't we scientifically-trained docs dish out a back-rub and a little Mozart with our precious prescriptions?

Although I was only with him for a few hours, and was thus not able to get into a long, detailed dialogue with him about his philosophy of medicine, I sense that Cable understands that a doctor's role is to help provide patients with a good life by treating a whole person — instead of merely *preventing* a miserable life by narrowly treating a physical ailment with drugs, the more common approach in medicine. Where is it written that only medication prescriptions improve a patient's quality of life, or that we should be embarrassed by wanting to help patients relax? I'm certain that there are a lot of patients out there whose pain is amplified by the crappy circumstances of their lives, because I've seen them and described them in the previous pages. It seems to me that, if we want to prevent pain, we have an obligation to help patients relax by any means necessary, and not just hand them a pill.

My guess is that there's a ton of docs out there that would snort at these suggestions. But we physicians marginalize guys like Cable at our peril.

Oncology
Friday, December 1

I spent two weeks looking for something to write about; today is the last day of the rotation, and I've come up empty-handed. I spent two weeks working mostly with the radiation oncologists, people who treat tumors by zapping them with gamma rays and whatnot. As a result, there were lots of people with brain tumors, facial tumors, and neck tumors—places where it's very tough for surgeons to go mucking about. I also spent an afternoon here and there with surgical oncologists checking out people who had their colons or rectums, or breasts, or lungs or arms removed to "cure" some cancer.

Mostly, though, what I did was walk in and out of exam rooms all day long following my doctor-du-jour. It became pretty clear early on that most of the doctors were at their happiest when I was at my silentest, and they regarded my normally inquisitive manner as being seriously annoying. I had little doubt that nobody would have noticed if I didn't show up to two, three, or four clinics in a row. Unfortunately, due to some quirk from my childhood where I must have gotten busted in a profound way for showing up five minutes late to dinner, I am apparently unable to blow off situations like these, fearing that I will be reprimanded and punished. Reprimanded? Punished? Hell, my guess is that if I no-showed at a few of these clinics I might well have been *thanked*! Still, I came, and the contribution of the past two weeks on my medical education were, approximately, nil.

They did give me a nice textbook on clinical oncology for free, though.

Radiology

Monday, December 4

Today, we were introduced to the course director, Dr. Meeghan. If Meeghan is at all representative of radiologists, it's going to be a fascinating two weeks. He entered into the lecture room at five minutes past 9 a.m. wearing Groucho Marx glasses with matching mustache, pacing back and forth, saying that he was late, which was something we had better get used to. "You know, this course used to be known as the radiation vacation, but you're going to discover that the medical school has raised the bar for you guys. Now I call it the clerkship from hell." Then he asked us a question.

"You guys know about that saying about history and physical being important?"

Everyone indicated they did. Since the beginning of our second year, when we began learning the basics of physical exam and taking a detailed patient history, we had been told repeatedly that "the history and physical will account for 80 percent of the diagnosis."

"Yeah, once upon a time I also used to think that bullshit about history and physical was true," Meeghan said. "But you're going to learn that pretty much *we're* the people making the diagnoses around the medical center these days."

Monday, December 11

Everyone went over together today to Children's Hospital for a peek at pediatric radiology. Pediatric radiology is an entire field unto itself, and requires a fellowship after the radiology residency. Because Children's Hospital is loaded with money, the radiology conference room is not only more plush than its brother over at the University, but it is also super high-tech. An entire wall is devoted to serving as a large screen, enabling the radiologists to pull up ten-foot high pictures of x-rays, MRIs, and CTs of children not greater than two or three feet in real-life length. It's an impressive facility.

The morning lecture consisted of looking at various kiddie x-rays, the most depressing of which were so-called "Silverman series" x-rays. The Silverman series is a head-to-toe set of x-rays used to detect child abuse. Since child abuse victims often have one or many occult fractures (that is, ones only apparent on x-ray), any child with an unusual fracture undergoes a Silverman series. The attending radiologist commented that these were not such a rare occurrence at Children's Hospital.

At lunch, one of the pediatric fellows brought us to a conference room while we ate (compliments of the department) to tell us about the career opportunities in peds radiology. I doubt that many of us there were truly considering radiology, much less radiology with kids, but the name of the game is to listen to the schpiel while you eat free food. All in all, it's not a bad deal. For about thirty minutes, you sit back and try to imagine yourself as Joe Doctor, Radiology Attending. Then, at the end, you realize that it isn't really an image that you like and you go back to whatever your original plans were.

Still, he pitched as hard as he could. He noted that radiologists generally can take vacation without having to worry about a specific patient or group of patients, that call isn't as brutal as it is for docs in primary care, and that the hours weren't anywhere near as long as most other specialties, though things have been getting worse in that respect.

"You all probably want to know what kind of money radiologists make when they get out," he said. This was true, but nobody was going to be that blunt about it and ask straightaway. "Well, the *mean* level for pediatric radiologists in the US for their first year out of fellowship is about two-hundred seventy nine thousand dollars. Now that's the mean, of course. If you're living in a place where most doctors want to live, somewhere warm and dry, say, like San Diego or Phoenix, then it's probably going to be lower, because managed care companies know that if you don't think you're being compensated well enough, there's five other people behind you who will be only too happy to take the job."

Two seventy-nine is well over double what the average pediatrician, internist, or family doc makes in private practice. My guess is that this very high figure is due to the cutback in radiology training programs in the past ten to fifteen years. Radiology *used* to be a very noncompetitive field, a bit like anesthesia these days. Since the cutbacks, the demand has grown for radiologists, and their salaries have become quite handsome in the past several years, which is why (in addition to the light call and limited patient responsibilities) it has become such a popular field.

"But if you go somewhere where there's a real demand for radiologist, and peds radiologists especially, you can find yourself making considerably more," he continued. "There are some places in the central Midwest that are so in need of good radiologists that, if you're willing to hustle and work six days a week, within a couple of years you can be making from seven to eight hundred thousand dollars a year."

That perked everyone up real quick.

One of the big downsides, he warned us, was that radiologists had extremely high malpractice insurance rates. We gave him confused looks. Why would radiologists, who generally don't perform any invasive procedures, get sued so much?

"Oh, that's easy," he said. "You'll look at some chest x-ray that says, 'rule out pneumonia' or something like that. So you'll take a look at the film, and you can be pretty careful looking at it, and you write a report that says it's a clear film. Then, six months later, the guy has a tumor in his lung, and when you know the location you go back and look at the film and, sure enough, you notice something very subtle. So some malpractice lawyer gets hold of that information and asks you in court, 'So, doctor, didn't you *see* the abnormality on the x-ray? It's right there,' and he can make it sound pretty convincing that it was clear as day in retrospect. There are too many opportunities for you to make errors like that."

XXXXXXXXX

If you've ever taken a close look at an x-ray film, you'll know that other than air, which is solid black, and bone or metal, which is solid white, that all other substances are various shades of gray. Looking at a mammogram (the x-ray film of breast tissue that is used in screening for breast cancer) can be daunting, in this respect. Breast tissue often appears to be a kind of light-grayish haze. The problem is that breast cancer doesn't look significantly different from normal tissue. The chapter I read in the radiology textbook would show a picture of a normal mammogram and one in which the patient had cancer, and I'd look at it and think, "Okay, what's different?" Obviously I'm no expert, but even as a beginner this task seemed orders of magnitude more difficult than finding a tumor on a CT scan.

I got a confirmation of this notion when the pediatric radiology fellow was talking to us about the job he'll be taking when he finishes his fellowship. He's going to work in a mid-size practice in Pennsylvania—a practice large enough to allow some specialization but small enough that he's still mostly a generalist. "I told them I'd be happy to do anything except mammography, which is fine, since they've got plenty of other people who are willing to do that," he said.

"Why do you want to avoid mammography?" someone asked.

"Because it's like trying to find a snowball in a blizzard," he replied.

Friday, December 15

Six months have gone by, the radiation vacation is over, and now the *real* vacation begins. For the first time since I walked corridors of Christ hospital in early July, I will have some time off to spend with my wife, hang out, read a book, party with my friends, and watch some flicks.

Radiology, despite Doc Meeghan's warnings about this being a clerkship from hell, turned out to be only slightly more engaging than my two weeks in oncology. Most of the time I sat around watching people read films. Every now and then I'd ask a question, and depending on which attending I was working for that day, I'd get a response. Most of the time it was fairly clear that answering lots of questions weren't high on the priority list of the attendings, so I ended up spending most of the past week seeking out Dr. Wang, a man perfectly willing to teach. This caused some friction with the department secretary by the end of the week, since the course requirements are to attend someplace *different* every day during the second week, but there was safety in numbers: Virtually everyone spent the week holed up in their place of choice. It's not like they were going to fail us, after all — we showed up, at least.

The presentation this morning was something of a debacle. When the two attendings who were evaluating us walked in, one said, "Okay, guys, let's make this as quick and painless as possible. Nobody go over five minutes, allright?"

For me, this was going to present a problem. Earlier last week I ran into a classmate who had taken radiology a few months back, and she had informed me that the presentations were to be approximately *fifteen* minutes in length. I had something on the order of twenty slides in my Power Point presentation, each practically bursting with information. How on earth was I going to cut corners?

"So, Doctor, um…Hatch, is it? What's the topic of your talk?" Dr. Balim asked.

"Radiographic presentations of connective-tissue disease, sir."

"Oh, that sounds very interesting."

Now, this is just a wild guess, but my suspicion is that he was *less* interested when, so Andrea informs me, I finished my final slide just about, um, seventeen minutes after that moment. "Jesus, Steven!" Andrea said afterward at lunch. "There must have been five of us that were trying to gesture to you to speed it up!"

"That *was* speeded up, girl," I said seriously in reply.

After lunch we took our final test of the front half of the year. Figuring that the class that I had thought I had taken was called "radiology," and figuring that radiology involved something called "looking at pictures," I naturally spent one or two hours each day over the past two weeks looking at chest and abdomen films, assuming that we would be tested on the basics of x-rays, CTs, MRIs, angiography, and maybe an image or two of ultrasound.

Silly me. You'd think after taking the first hundred or so tests that I would have realized that the only kind of test apparently given in this medical center is in the question-and-four-possible-answer format. Instead of being asked if I could identify the lingular lobe on a chest film, I was instead asked about what kinds of radio-opaque dyes are most likely associated with an allergic response. There was not one image out of fifty questions. Not one. I needed thirty questions to pass, and I deeply suspect it's going to be a close call.

But as long as I pass, I won't make any bones about it, as it were. My only goal throughout the electives has been to get by. If it holds me back from a research career at the NIH, so be it. Somehow, I don't think selection committees are going to turn me down if I couldn't cut it for two weeks in radiology.

That said, today I passed the halfway mark. Now it's Miller Time.

<u>five</u>

the Big Three begins:

kiddos

Tuesday, January 9

The three interns on my team (the "green" team—the hospital is divided into different-colored teams based on subspecialty: The "purple" team is neurology, the "silver" team handles pulmonary and gastrointestinal cases, we of the green are a bit of a catch-all) are on a retreat, and so rounds today consisted of the two senior residents, Art and Scott, going over the caseloads with the attending, Dr. Harlan. The atmosphere was jocular, with Art and Scott having jokes for every case that was discussed. One that caused particular hilarity concerned a patient named "Kiss," a late adolescent who had been severely mentally retarded since he was run over by a truck at an early age. The joking didn't have much to do with the patient, but rather his name, which they insisted writing in lettering similar to the rock band Kiss (with the Nazi-looking lettering for the two S's) on the dry-marker case-management board. This was the source of great mirth between Art and Scott for several minutes, as was a patient named Willis, whom they referred to privately as "What you talkin' about, Willis?" after the phrase made famous by Gary Coleman on the TV show *Different Strokes*.

The rounds (which, like psych rounds, are done away from the patients and in a sort-of conference room) took only a half-hour and that's the last of Dr. Harlan that we saw for the rest of the day. Art and Scott indicated that that's about how often we'll see her. As a rule, it doesn't sound like the attendings have much to do with the minutiae of case management. They like to know what's going on when a patient is first admitted, and then as the diagnoses are narrowed down and the treatment plan is put into effect, they let the residents manage the interns, who in turn execute the plays.

As we finished, Scott mentioned that they ought to assign cases to us students. "You're right," said Art, and immediately suggested one of the teenagers with cystic fibrosis should be assigned to one of us.

Scott looked at him crossly. "You don't want to give them CF patients, do you?"

"Why not?"

"Oh, man, they're so nasty. Don't let's start them there."

"Yeah, I guess you're right. But they *should* have to deal with a CF case before they leave here."

"Yeah, of course," said Scott. Then he added to us, "CF patients are pretty miserable. They've been in and out of this hospital their entire lives. They know the hospital better than you or I ever could. They resent that, and they resent us. So you'll walk by their doors, and they'll have written, 'Don't wake me up before ten o'clock AM,' or, 'NO—I DON'T want you to listen to my lungs today!' and so we don't want to start you with something like that. They can be pretty rough."

We divvied up a few cases each. I was thinking about asking for this girl with anorexia nervosa since I've never worked with an anorexic and it sounded like an interesting challenge, but my classmate Avital beat me to the punch. Then I realized that she wants to go into child psychiatry, and so obviously this girl was the perfect case for her. My two cases include a 9 year-old who has just got diagnosed with diabetes, and an 18 year-old with severe mental retardation and cerebral palsy who had a spinal fusion surgery a month ago and now can't seem to hold any food down. Our docs originally thought she might have a problem called "superior mesenteric artery syndrome," which means that her blood supply to her guts were being squeezed off, making her unable to absorb nutrition. But they did a barium swallow down in radiology, and they concluded that her arterial supply was fine. When I went to see her today and introduce myself to her mother, she was throwing up food that her mother had just tried to feed to her. So, regardless of the fact that we were able to "rule out" the SMA syndrome, the girl's no better off.

Thursday, January 11

The interns returned from their retreat yesterday, and so I think the business of learning on the job will begin in earnest.

Because the interns were away at a retreat the past three days, the four students haven't had much guidance from Art and Scott, both of whom have been very busy trying to cover for the work of their missing interns. So the schedule during Tuesday and Wednesday was filled with morning rounds lasting about two hours, a one-hour period to write chart notes, a radiology conference, a noontime teaching session with Dr. Archibald Boone (the course director) and then we took off, since there wasn't anything else that we were clearly supposed to do.

The intern that I'm going to be working with most closely is Trina Kim because she shares my call schedule every fourth night. I start tomorrow night, which will mean that tomorrow I'll be getting new patients and doing their workups—a "workup" being a history and physical exam, ordering the necessary labs to arrive at an accurate diagnosis and the meds to ensure adequate treatment. This is the part of medicine that I think is fun, because each patient is something like a mystery and how we do the history, physical, and tests will reveal the plot.

In addition to getting the interns back, we met with the pharmacologist this morning so that she could give us a taste-test of many of the common medications that we prescribe for the kids. She had several vials of the meds, and we would squirt about two drops of medication onto our plastic spoons, and bottoms up! We'd wash it down with a little grape kool-aid and graham crackers, and take on the next med. The amount that we were taking in was pretty harmless, and she had to remind us more than once that whatever we were tasting was being administered to the children in a significantly higher dose. "I've never had anyone get sick on me yet while doing this exercise," she said cheerily as we began.

Cheer was probably necessary since we began with the various oral preparations of prednisone, an immune-suppressing steroid that is most commonly used for severe asthmatics who have been hospitalized. We took three different samples of prednisone, each equally as nasty as the other. If you've never had the pleasure of taking oral prednisone, it is the worst punishment you could administer to your taste buds. It doesn't taste simply bad; it's a Hiroshima on your tongue. I can't describe it except to say that the flavor doesn't hit you until you've already swallowed the medicine, that its taste is part metallic, part vomit, and (undoubtedly the worst part) that it doesn't easily wash out, but instead lingers for several minutes.

After the second steroid, Avital looked somewhat pale and decided to throw in the towel. We had fourteen others to get through. I thought about giving her grief for so easily quitting, especially since the point of the exercise was to learn what the kids *had* to go through, but I kept my mouth shut and she left the room not long after.

By that point we had managed to endure a few other truly yucky meds, including a potassium-supplement preparation that tasted like salty clam juice that had been sitting out all day in the hot summer sun. The ibuprofen and acetaminophen liquids weren't too bad, and eventually we managed to reach the shores of tastiness with the antibiotics, of all things, nearly all of which were pleasant to sample. Amoxicillin was the big winner, with a smooth bubble-gum taste (several of the antibiotics, despite tasting good, had the grittiness of sandpaper) and a bright neon-pink color to boot. Even so, the memory of the prednisone was so overwhelming it was difficult to enjoy the session much, and we sampled the last med almost forty-five minutes after the first ones.

As we were about to leave, the pharmacist looked into her bag and then looked at me. "Oh, I *do* have it," she said to me. "I know you were joking, but I really do have the liquid haldol if you'd like to try it."

I chuckled. "Hey, if you got it, why shouldn't I give it a spin? How 'bout you, Michael?" So my classmate Michael and I sat there and taste-tested one of the most potent antipsychotic medications available. It actually had the most neutral taste of everything I tried, just a bit more viscous than water and the slightest bit salty.

Saturday, January 13

First night of call last night. I got a good amount of sleep — about 4 hours. One of the new admissions was a 12 year-old kid from Charleston, West Virginia who had been having recurrent pneumonias, and was finally bronchoscoped (a TV camera stuck down his lungs) here in Cincinnati, where a pen cap was found hanging out in his lower right lung and removed. Word to the masses: Breathing in pen caps can have deleterious consequences. This kid will be on intravenous antibiotics for the next month.

So at several points during the night I call up my resident, Trina, to see if she needs help, can I pick up any new patients, et cetera, and she tells me each time that I don't need to pick up anyone new but just stay with the patients that I had been following and do some reading about their conditions should I see fit. By nine-thirty I was done with any responsibilities that I had toward the patients, so I sat down at the computer and did a literature search on foreign-body aspiration to present a paper the following morning. I also did a lit search on orbital cellulitis (an infection of the soft tissues around and within the eye socket) since the other new patient I had picked up that night had come in with his left eye swollen shut. After I read the articles, I hunkered down in my call room until about 1:30 and decided to call it a night.

The call rooms at Children's — at least those for the med students — aren't very pleasant. Two people sleep in them on bunk beds, and they're about as large as a walk-in closet. You can't actually enter the room and step right in, but instead you have to shimmy your way in-between the bed and the lone chair to the left of the doorway, then close the door, and then move into the five- or six-square feet of free space in the room. It makes changing out of your day-clothes and into your scrubs a unique challenge. And once I took my shoes off (after having been walking all over the hospital for about sixteen hours), I knew that the stench had no way of quickly dissipating, so I hoped that whoever came to the room that night came several hours later.

When I got up to the room, another student had staked a claim on the lower bed by laying his bookbag across it, which left me with the upper bunk. Once I was tucked in, I had about two feet of clearance above my head until I hit the ceiling, and the bed rocked to and fro if I moved even slightly. Great, I thought, this is going to be a really fun month of calls. I fell asleep, and later awoke when Jason Argyle, another one of the older students who was working the purple team, came in at about 2:30. He said, "Oh, that was your bag?"

"Which one?" I asked.

"That silver one on the top bunk. I thought it was Alex's."

"You've got to be kidding me. There's a third person who's coming to this room?"

"I don't know. Guess we'll find out soon enough."

And we did find out about an hour later, after I had managed to fall asleep peacefully a second time, when Alex did come into the room (sound of door opening, shuffling feet moving to the open space, door closing, lights going on). Alex looked pretty shocked to see two people asleep in his call room. The three of us looked at each other trying to figure out, first, how on earth nobody managed to notice this problem earlier, and second, what we were going to do about it at three-thirty. Alex was gentlemanly about it and said that he'd just check back in with his resident and explain the situation and either find a bed somewhere in the hospital or just go home.

I got up this morning and visited my patients, all geared up to give my first real presentation. I wondered if the regular attending, Dr. Harlan, would be there, since this was a weekend day. She was. Presenting a patient is not only the bread-and-butter of what almost every practicing physician does on a near-daily basis, but it's one of the major educational goals for the third-year student—perhaps *the* educational goal. Being able to present a patient well is one of the biggest keys to success during the Big Three, so I was eager to make a good first impression on Harlan. I figured that I'd sail through the presentation, casually toss out my references to the journal articles that I had read last night, and let the residents carry on with the rest of rounds.

A presentation is, when done properly, roughly a five-minute account about the patient. Presentations have all the basic structure of a short story in essence, with a beginning, middle, and end; the content involves the vocabulary of scientific specialists, but the form is pure narrative.

This is a very basic idea of how one sounds:

"Sally is a thirteen year-old female who has complaints of abdominal pain. She began to feel this pain—a vague, diffuse pain in her epigastric region—when she woke up this morning. She remained home from school, where she began to run a fever of 101 degrees. She denies chills, nausea, vomiting, diarrhea, or vaginal discharge. By late afternoon, she developed intense pain in her right lower quadrant, and was driven by her mother to the Emergency Department.

"Past medical history is significant only for mild exercise-induced asthma and for tonsillectomy at age six. She takes albuterol for rescue therapy for the asthma, and has no known drug allergies. Family medical history is non-contributory, with no family members suffering from inflammatory bowel disease. Social history is that she lives with her mother, father, and two brothers, twins age eight. She denies smoking, alcohol or drug consumption, or sexual activity.

"Physical exam revealed a young woman in moderate distress with guarding. Vitals were heart rate 88, blood pressure of 102 over 75, respiratory rate of 16, and temp of 102.2 degrees. Heart was regular rate and rhythm, lungs were clear to auscultation bilaterally. Abdominal exam showed intense pain in the right lower quadrant with maximum pain at McBurney's point and rebound tenderness. No masses were appreciated and bowel sounds were present. Pelvic exam was normal. Cranial nerves were intact. Pupils were equal round, reactive to light and showed accommodation. The rest of the exam was within normal limits. Labs showed no serum electrolyte abnormalities; CBC showed a white blood cell count of 16.5 with a left shift; serum amylase and lipase were normal, as were liver function tests. Beta-HCG was negative. Abdominal ultrasound failed to show any abnormalities."

At this point, you take a breath, because you're hitting your conclusion. Any third-year med student will know what's coming, and probably a lot of lay people can recognize this as well.

"Assessment is a thirteen year-old female with signs and symptoms consistent with acute appendicitis. The plan is to consult surgery for immediate resection either via laparotomy or preferably laparoscopy. I also hope to rule-out inflammatory bowel disease, tubo-ovarian abscess, or pelvic inflammatory disease."

That's the flavor for what it's like. You tell the care team what the patient showed up with to the hospital or office (their "chief complaint"), when things started to go wrong for the patient (the "history of present illness"), and then give pertinent information that might be related to their treatment this time around. Then you explain what you found on exam and the lab test results. By that point, if you've presented it well, when you state your assessment, everyone should have a very good sense of what is going on.

When you see a presentation done like this, you also can understand why it's a medical dictum that "history and physical will give you 80 percent of the information you need to know."* The fancy-science part of medicine (labs, imaging, biopsies and whatnot) really only serves to confirm what the history indicates. Say you present a boy with a three-month history of progressively worsening neurological symptoms including seizures, inability to move his right arm, and a difficulty understanding what people are saying to him. You still *need* to do an MRI to find out what's going on, but odds are that he's got a tumor over in the left side of his head, because the presentation — the story — suggests it.

So I went to present my patients for what was really the first time since I began third year. You see, surgery presentations aren't taken very seriously and I presented maybe four or five times, and then only to the residents. I didn't do any presentations in family medicine or in any of the electives; and in psych I did several presentations, but they were characteristically psych

---

* Not, as you'll recall, that some radiologists agree with this sentiment.

presentations, where the emphasis was less on physical exam and labs but rather on their psychiatric state.

I can't tell you how well I performed. Dr. Harlan has a very energetic persona, and she often interrupts with questions to clarify. So after awhile it became hard to tell how well I presented since I stopped and started so often. She isn't obviously critical—in fact, she's usually very encouraging. That may seem good, but in terms of knowing how she's going to evaluate me, it doesn't help at all. At any rate, after I finished discussing the boy of pen-cap removal fame, I said, "Yeah, and I was doing some reading last night of a case report of the same thing in Italy. It was almost exactly the same situation, and this kid's atelectasis [jargon for "sticky parts of lung"] was completely resolved a year later. The only difference between them and us was that they used steroids to treat him, but they admit that they don't know if it helped any." Then I read a few lines from the paper about the steroids.

As soon as I finished I wanted to shrivel up. It came out so forced, so awkward-sounding, that I felt like I was Chief Sycophant at Med School U. The feeling was like, *well, here I am, guys, gunning for honors, and I just happened to be reading this journal article*...Worse yet, the response from Harlan was nothing more than a pleasant nod. If she had liked it, in theory she would have said, "Oh, that's interesting. Do you have a copy?" But no such luck for me.

Monday, January 15

Children's Hospital of Cincinnati has one of the largest genetics clinics in the country, and many of the patients walking the corridors on the lower levels of the hospital are bound for appointments with some of the specialists working in or around the field of genetics: The cranio-facial clinic, the metabolic disorders clinic, etc. If you pass these kids in the hallways, you'll see them with their siblings and parents, and you'll think, "there's something not quite right about that family," but you'd be hard pressed to say precisely *what* doesn't seem right.

"One thing that should make you suspect a possible chromosomal or genetic abnormality is the feeling that their facial features don't seem to add up right," said Dr. Boone today in our five-classmate teaching session. "If one of them strikes you as the proverbial 'FLK,' then you should think about a genetic workup."

We all looked at him. "What's an 'FLK'?" I asked.

"Oh, you've never heard of it? I forget that you guys are new to this. 'FLK' is short for 'Funny-Looking Kid.' I admit, it's a horribly insensitive term that's been used for decades by medical staff across the country. Genetics experts can tell many of the chromosomal disorders just by looking at a kid, but general pediatricians often have a harder time elucidating exactly what's wrong, so people just started referring to these patients as 'FLKs.' Of course, *never* write that on any official document, because that's an instant lawsuit that you'll certainly lose. It's happened in the past."

Wednesday, January 17

Call night with Trina was not one of the better experiences I've had. Everything we tried to say to each other came out awkward. Early yesterday afternoon, I needed to page Trina to explain to her that I needed to go home from call for about an hour. I had to go home because my wife Miriam and I have been having problems conceiving, and for the first time in several months we knew that Miriam was ovulating as she had just come from the obstetrician, who recommended that we get a baby-making session in ASAP just in case that little egg was about to get on the loose.

Obviously this was information that I didn't want to share with Trina, much less anyone else in the medical center. Thus, all I should have said to Trina was, "I have some personal business that I must take care of. I'll be gone for about an hour, and I'll get back as soon as I can," and left it at that.

But here's how the conversation actually played out. Trina returns my page.

"Hello, Trina?"

"Yes."

"It's Steven. There's a favor I need to ask. I'm going to need to go home for about an hour tonight. I don't know if you want to know why, but I've got a real humdinger of a reason." I gave an uncomfortable chuckle.

"Sure. Why do you need to go?"

"*Ummm*, well, you see..." and off I went.

Later on in the evening, when I had caught up to Trina and met with a new patient, Trina pulled me aside to try to be encouraging. "Listen, I know how hard it is to be in your third year, when you've got all kinds of responsibility and you don't have time for family and personal concerns, so don't feel like you can't leave if you need to. It's okay for you just to tell me that there's some personal business that you need to attend to." Then she paused, started to add something, laughed nervously, and said, "Yeah, that's it." Like she was about to say, "I *really* didn't need to know all that."

• • • • • • • •

Senior resident Scott Sullivan's sense of humor: A fourth-year medical student from Georgia was spending the day in the hospital for a "second look." It's a little dance that fourth-years do for programs they are eager to attend. You apply, and if you're good enough to get an interview, you visit a first time in the late fall or early winter. Then, before the Match, you can stroke the program a bit if you come back out to take a second look. In theory it heightens your chances, because programs like to give high ranks to people who in turn rank them #1 — this enhances the program's prestige, theoretically. I have no idea if it works in practice but many who can afford the plane ticket do it.

Anyway, this student struck up a conversation with the other senior, Art, as we were walking toward the Wednesday radiology conference. Avital, Scott and I were walking a little ahead of them, chatting about nothing in particular. Avital craned her neck back to eavesdrop on their conversation. Then she caught back up with us with an incredulous look.

"They're talking about their *MCAT* scores," she said with equal parts ridicule and surprise. MCAT scores, those needed to get into med school, don't play a very important part of residency considerations. It's like talking about how you did on your SATs when you are applying to law school.

"Well, it's no longer considered polite to drop your pants in public," Scott responded. Meaning: To check to see who's got the bigger dick for bragging rights.

Also included in Scott's repertoire are his morning observations during rounds. One morning we were discussing a baby that weighed 10 kilograms — way, way above the normal range for a kid his age. Stacy, one of the interns, said, "I saw him one morning when I was rounding, and he was gobbling something up, and I said to the mother, 'Oh, he's having breakfast now, I can come back later,' and she said, 'Breakfast? Aw, he had breakfast hours ago. This is just a *snack!*'"

"We better not put him in the same room as the other infant we're covering. He might eat *him* for a snack," Scott said. "We'll stop by for a check-up, look around and wonder, *now where is the baby?*, and then see a leg coming out of his mouth as he belches. Not a good idea."

• • • • • • • • •

Senior resident Art Pollack's sense of humor: There are three buildings that house patients in the Children's Medical Center. The new building is known as the Tower and will eventually be the main hospital building when the construction is completed; we do most of our work in what is called simply the "Hospital," a building that will be torn down when the new hospital is built; and then there is the Pavilion, a Stalinist-style building that is removed from everything else and houses only a few wards.

The Pavilion is not only geographically remote, its layout isn't very conducive to great critical care. The nursing stations don't sit in the middle of the ward, as they do on all other floors, but rather in a tucked-away spot in which half of the rooms are out of view. But there also seems to be something about the nursing over there that makes some of the house staff queasy. Orders are written by the residents but sometimes can take hours to be acted upon; patients don't get their vital signs checked as often as they should; and in general, the nurses don't communicate well to the house staff. The residents were complaining about all these things at the end of rounds today.

"If I knew that my kids needed to go to the hospital, and they told me that they were going to the Pavilion, I'd take them out of the hospital," Art said matter-of-factly. "They'd get just as good a treatment at home. In fact, I think probably the only good thing about the Pavilion is that it's located right next to a major medical center."

This caused much mirth among the tired and overwrought interns.

Sunday, January 21   post-call

Medical students during their first two years spend most of their time sitting in front of a book reading about diseases and drugs. Residents spend most of their time learning how to treat patients and become adept at clinical diagnosis. In between are us, the third- and fourth-year med students, who spend a good deal of time posing for their superiors while transitioning from diseases in books to diseases in real patients. Most of the time I feel like I'm not learning very much, and I become very scared that, in approximately 18 months, I'm going to be entrusted with keeping very sick people alive. But every now and again, I get a glimpse of the bigger picture, and I'm able, if only for fleeting moments, to see the beauty of medicine — not just being able to diagnose diseases, but being able to make a plan, follow patients, and see them through to health.

Last night's call was one of those moments, and it's also the first time in the two weeks where I felt like Trina and I managed to get into some sort of a rhythm together, leaving behind the awkwardness that's been plaguing the two of us. It was a very quiet afternoon, and during this time I didn't see her very much. It was snowing outside, maybe two inches, and the hospital was very quiet. According to resident lore, when it snows on weekends, admissions drop: Parents seem to feel that their kids, no matter how sick, can wait until the beginning of the week before they see the doctor.

So I told Trina that I was going to go meet with Andrea to work on questions for our discussion group, and that *as soon* as we picked up a new admission, could she please page me? I told her that I would go and check up on a baby with bronchiolitis that we picked up overnight, and I'd be waiting for her page, and we'd touch base in a few hours at most.

Hours passed and I hadn't heard from her. I was getting pissed, thinking that we had gotten new admissions and she wasn't letting me at them. What was I going to do come tomorrow, when I needed to present a patient? Finally I broke down and paged her at about 2:30. I told her about the baby I saw, a little three-monther who wasn't rallying very well despite some oxygen therapy. He didn't look especially sick, but he did look especially zonked. We agreed to go meet at his room. I figured it would take five or ten minutes, and I'd be back working on the questions with Andrea.

When we got to the kid, Trina was concerned. Mom had removed the nasal cannula feeding the oxygen ("he doesn't like it on," said the mother). We asked how much milk he had been drinking (about half his normal amount) and urinating (not very much). Trina looked at the mother and said, "I really think we need to get an IV in him and get some fluids into him right away, so I'm going to write an order to get that done, okay?"

Mom looked at her somewhat cross-eyed and I instantly knew that there was going to be a problem. "Are you *sure* that he needs an IV?" she asked. "I *really* don't want my baby stuck. They were trying to get an IV in earlier, and it must have taken an hour and he was in agony. I'm not going through that again." Tears started to well up in her eyes.

Trina gave her best sympathetic look and very gently said, "It must be very hard to watch your son in any pain. But the truth is that he'll be in less pain over the long run if we get some fluids into him now. He'll bounce back much quicker."

"But he's *been* feeding!" she protested.

Her friend who was there to visit chimed in, "Yeah. Doesn't *milk* count as fluids?"

Trina didn't look it but I could tell that she was not interested in having a battle with mom about this, and was trying to figure out the best way to get around this impasse. "It's true that he's feeding, but he's not getting enough. I know that this must be very hard, but you've got to try to trust us to help him get better. He really needs fluids. I've got to go now, but I'll stop by later, okay?" I stayed in the room a few extra minutes to try to let the mom vent a little bit, figuring that some good-cop, bad-cop would make her feel understood. She wasn't quite hysterical, and she was going along with the plan, albeit reluctantly.

When I got outside, Trina was obviously nonplussed. She flung her arms in slight exasperation and said, "Steven, could you tell me *why* parents will bring their kid to a major medical center, and then not let us treat them? I mean, if we don't give him IV fluids and oxygen, what are we doing for him that couldn't be done at home?"

"Yeah," I answered. "I really liked her friend. We're halfway there with the mom and then she starts in. I wanted to smack her."

Anyway, the order got written, and about two hours later one of the nurses, a guy named TR, put in the IV line. Thank God (to say nothing of thanking TR) the stick went well on the first time out. Several hours later, TR informed me, the boy was happy as a lark, playing with his grandparents who had come to visit.

But my work with Trina had just begun. We proceeded back over to the Hospital (we were in the Pavillion section) where we had to deal with an emergency — two, actually — and for the first time I felt like Trina was willing to rely on me for help. The first problem was a kid with Down Syndrome who was in the hospital, also with bronchiolitis. Trina was "cross-covering" a patient normally seen by an intern on another team who was taking the weekend day off. Interns basically hope nothing goes wrong with cross-cover patients, but in this case, nothing seemed to be working *right*. The kid was vomiting up her food, and her breathing was labored. Mom was a bit stressed, especially since the plan apparently was for discharge, and mom didn't think she was ready to be discharged, especially since she hadn't been seen by the doctor who had been following her up until that point.

I didn't say very much, and when Trina's pager went off in mid-conversation with mother, I just held out my hand and Trina turned to me and handed it off. When I answered the page, I was talking to a psychiatry nurse who wanted to know if the medical consult that had been requested was going to come. I fetched Trina, and when Trina took the call, I learned that Trina had been called about an hour ago about this depressed teenager who had been admitted and was looking pretty bad. Her blood pressure was eighty over twenty, which is *really* not very good. Trina told the nurse to get an IV in her as soon as possible and she would be there shortly. The hour had passed, and when Trina hadn't shown, the nurse got concerned.

"Well, when did she get the IV fluids?" Trina asked. Based on what I heard next, the nurse must have indicated that she had not *yet* received the IV. Trina raised her voice for the first time I had seen in two weeks. "I don't think you understand. This is an *emergency*! We've got to get fluids in her *now*!" She looked around, with a look like *what next?* and I told her I'd go down and take care of it. Whether or not I could was an open question, but I thought I'd give it a go. Couldn't have hurt, given the state of things.

I got down, saw the girl, whose blood pressure was holding steady at 80/50 but we wanted to get things taken care of pronto. "I called Central Booking four times," the nurse said. "You think you can do better, by all means please call them."

I called Central Booking and asked them what the problem was. "Oh, the person who's supposed to get the IV over to you, her pager wasn't working. She's on her way."

"Is she on her way *now*?"

"Yeah."

"No. I mean is she physically walking towards us right at

this moment? Otherwise I'm coming there to get the equipment. We can't wait any longer. We've already waited too long."

"She is on her way, right now. Thank you." Click.

Went back up and told Trina that we had temporarily put the fire out, and I was going back down to witness them insert the IV. By the time I got there, another psych nurse was doing the insertion. I held the kid's hand and told her that she'd be okay. Which was true, but not of much help. She looked pretty miserable. I do not look forward to my first IV insertion when the time comes. That is, as a *patient*. I pity the patient that's my first IV stick.

By the time Trina and I hooked up an hour later (throwing-up-baby problem taken care of), she was clearly grateful for the help I had provided. Suddenly I felt as if I almost might enjoy the final stretch with her. Maybe even learn something, too.

• • • • • • • • •

My classmate Dirk Jablonski said that his favorite part of working at Children's was that he'd go down to the child activity center and get on the Sony PlayStation with his patients and play them when he had a spare hour to kill. He'd always lose, he said, not out of *noblesse oblige* but rather because he wasn't *capable* of winning. "They're brutal," he said. "They're better than you could ever hope to be. Still, it was a blast playing anyway."

What is my favorite perk of being on call at Children's?

Sometime between midnight and one, when I've finished writing my notes on the patients, but before I sit down and do an hour or two of reading about their conditions, I head onto the floor. On each wing of each floor is a little kitchenette, and it has a refrigerator stocked with various juices and goodies for the children. I cruise on over to the kitchenette, open up the fridge, and pull out two pint-size chocolate milk cartons — the kind I used to drink as a grade-schooler. Then I go to the charge station, and bask in the silence of the hospital at that hour, guzzling down that syrupy chocolate concoction, and feel a little like a kid again.

It's awesome. The night nurses think I'm completely nuts, but I love it.

Tuesday, January 23   pre-call

Today in rounds, Trina was talking about dealing with some overanxious parents whose child was grunting and grimacing when he had bowel movements. Apparently, they were very nearly beside themselves when discussing their child's problem, concluding that he had some sort of gastrointestinal disorder. Trina managed to observe one of these episodes, and after careful inspection of the stool in the diaper, in addition to obtaining the labs and a thorough medical history of the child, had concluded that, at least in terms of his bowel movements, there was nothing out of the ordinary. She had tried to reassure the parents, but to no avail.

Scott Sullivan, himself a father, got slightly irritated as he heard this. "What's the matter with these people? *All* babies grunt and strain and grimace when they have a bowel movement," he said.

"Hey, so do I," Art Pollack offered. "Give him a Sports Illustrated. It works for me."

Saturday, January 27   pre-call

Wednesday night I picked up four new kids, and all of them except one are gone today. That's not such a big deal because I have today off — my first full day off in two weeks — and consequently I'm not at the hospital with nothing to do, but still it feels like it's hard to do learning about my patients when they're in the door and out the door in record time.

Things did not used to be this way. I'm not capable of giving a detailed history of hospital stays in the United States, but I'm pretty confident in saying that, as little as fifteen to twenty years ago, a hospital stay for a kid with, say, bronchiolitis (a respiratory infection, one of the most common conditions we see on the green team) was much longer than it is now (as little as one or two days). From the standpoint of the patient and the family, this is often good, since they get back home to more intimate surroundings and a higher level of comfort. But as a medical student, patients become a blur, and you don't get to know your patients very well.

One of my patients is a 15 year-old with Cystic Fibrosis and is my first CFer. Since the Green Team is designed to handle the pulmonary cases, we get almost all the CFers in the hospital. He's a pretty active kid going through his *first* hospitalization, which is fairly astonishing for a CF patient. Most come to the hospital for the first time at a very early age, such as four or five, which begins a cycle that lasts throughout the course of their illness.

As you recall, our senior residents were somewhat reluctant to hand out CF cases to us during the first two weeks, despite the fact that it's the bread-and-butter of the Green Team. They wanted us to adjust to the flow of the hospital and become better acquainted with our roles as medical students before throwing us into the lions' den.

CFers are the most challenging cases in the hospital from a "social" management standpoint. First of all, many of the CF cases in the hospital are teenagers, and these CF teenagers are no different than any other teen in the sense that they want to be independent, and they especially don't want interference or help from adults. Second, as I noted earlier, most of these kids have been coming in and out of the hospital several times a year for more than a decade. They know the hospital better than anybody. Because of this acquired knowledge, they'll push you around, and tell *you* what you can or can't do. Most of the residents make compromises with them to keep peace and keep a hold on their own sanity.

These kids are by far the angriest kids in the hospital. They have a right to be. While they watch their schoolmates and playmates blossom and dream about what they're going to do with their lives, CFers cope with the grind of multiple hospitalizations. They also probably wonder if they will be able to live anything approaching a normal life for what little time they'll be able to live it, because only a small number of them will make it to thirty. A lot of them won't even be lucky enough to make it to twenty, depending on how you define "luck."

All in all, I figured that this kid was a good CF patient to pick up, since he hadn't yet acquired this hardened, wizened attitude. But a teenager's a teenager, and I realized after talking to him for awhile something that I had forgotten about myself for several years: I'm very awkward in front of teenagers. I find it exceedingly hard to relate to them, to chisel through that hard exterior and gain their trust.

When I walked in, Ted, my patient, was getting something called *chest physiotherapy*. It's a medieval form of medicine but it works. Since CF is a disease in which patients produce very thick mucous plugs in their lungs, one way to keep their lungs as clear as possible is to literally shake the chest up to loosen the mucus and cause the patient to cough it up. That used to be accomplished with a massage therapist, but the same thing is done with this chest physiotherapy contraption, which looks like a life preserver vest hooked up to a pump that rapidly cycles pulses of high-pressure air. It sounds a bit like a treadmill and it was utterly impossible for Ted to speak without his voice quavering all over the place. Which was fine; he was obviously not interested in giving his medical history for the fourth time today. So I talked mostly to his mother instead.

His story was unusual for CF and involves not one but two blown diagnoses. He was not diagnosed with CF until he was five, and the lag in diagnosis may have made his condition worse, although as I said above I've never heard of a CFer coming in for his first post-diagnosis hospitalization at age 15. (By contrast, there's a seven year-old on our service who has been in two to three times a year since *birth*.) Mother took Ted to see a man who had been *her* pediatrician. As an infant, he had been hospitalized twice at about 12 and 15 months with pneumonia.

Stop right there. *Any* medical student who's gone through pediatrics knows that two hospitalizations for pneumonia in a short time span, in the absence of a known cause, should prompt suspicion about CF, and the kid should probably get a sweat chloride test, the diagnostic test for CF. But, oddly, this pediatrician did not order the test, instead explaining that he had childhood asthma, and gave a referral to the local allergist.

In the meantime, Ted was having problems absorbing his food, and his stools had become very oily and fat-laden. This is another classic sign of CF, since the thick mucus caused by the disease also plugs up the pancreas, the organ responsible for producing chemicals that aid in fat and nutrient absorption among other things. The pediatrician *and* allergist both dismissed the unusual stools as a quirk, and told mom not to worry.

A year or two after this, in a case completely unrelated to Ted, the pediatrician had tried to perform a minor procedure on a kid in his office using a drug called *lidocaine*. There's nothing wrong with using the drug, but it's generally wise to do so with some resuscitation equipment around, since it can cause the heart to stop on rare occasion. This doc was not prepared for such a complication, and the kid died in the office. The pediatrician lost his license, causing Ted's mom to search for a new doc. They found a young new doc fresh out of residency. As she first met them and took Ted's medical history, she asked if he had been tested for CF, since it sounded suspicious. Mom said she didn't think so, that the doc had said he had asthma. The new doc asked her to check it with the allergist next time they saw him, because if not, she believed that Ted should get "sweated" — the pet name for taking the sweat chloride test — to make sure he didn't have CF.

The allergist was dismissive, and told Ted's mom that she was dealing with an overzealous and very young clinician; in short, the new doc didn't know what she was talking about. Mom repeated this story to the woman, who advised that, at the very least, he should be evaluated by a pediatric gastroenterologist for his unusual stools. The GI doc, in taking the history, asked the same question the new pediatrician posed: Has he been tested for CF? Again, the mother said he had not, and the doc said, well, he should get one. He did, and the test was positive. That was ten years ago, in 1990.

"I was so mad at that allergist, I called him up to tell him," Ted's mom told me. "I got his secretaries, you know, who wouldn't let me talk to him directly. They said, 'Can you tell me what this is about?' and I said that they had better put me on with him so that I can tell him he *failed* to diagnose my son with CF for four years! So he got on, and I let him have it." I thought that both the allergist and the now-defunct pediatrician were both very lucky that they weren't sued for malpractice. A baby with two pneumonias who produces oily and fatty stools? That's not a tricky presentation for CF; that's how they write "sample problem" clinical cases for third-year medical students. There are no complicated or confounding factors to throw you off the scent. It's a classic presentation. And not one, but two of them dropped the ball.

Anyway, since then, Ted's been doing about as well as a CFer can do in childhood. He's been as active as any other kid—playing on the baseball team, for instance—and, other than some nightly chest physiotherapy and an oxygen mask, has been spared the brunt of the constant medical interventions common for CF patients. This didn't change his disposition, though, which was understandably unenthusiastic at the outset of what might prove to be a week-long hospital admission. I vowed to get in, get the history, and get out as fast as possible.

After I finished getting the history from his mother, the physiotherapy pump machine finally stopped and Ted could talk, so I addressed the rest of my questions to him. "That must feel good to have that stop," I said. He stared back at me and said nothing. "So, how are you doing right now? Are you having any difficulty breathing?" He indicated no. "Are you feeling unusually tired?" He again shook his head. Just as I was about to ask him another question, the Halls lozenge that I had been sucking on to keep my cough suppressed slipped loose, dribbled right out of my mouth and onto the table on which I had been writing. Ted, who hadn't been looking directly at me throughout the interview, glanced sideways for a second or two, then returned to his off-in-the-distance gaze. Well, *that* must have looked impressive to mother and son, I thought. I'm going to have a spanking good time with this kiddo.

•••••••••

The second patient I picked up is Clark. Clark shouldn't be in the hospital. He's a seventeen year-old guy who came in with what may or may not have been a seizure. He was working at a local fast-food store, having what he described as a vicious migraine, and then he "passed out" for maybe twenty or thirty seconds. (I put it in quotes because those were his words and there apparently weren't witnesses to his passing out, so we don't know whether he had a seizure or he just doubled over in pain for half a minute.) His friends drove him to the Emergency Department, where he was evaluated and recommended for admission.

Why they admitted him is not clear. In the ED, he underwent a CT to rule out serious brain problems that might have caused this episode, such as a brain tumor or intracranial bleed. It was negative. He got an EKG to rule out any heart problems that might have caused him to faint, and it was negative. He also got a tox screen to check for the presence of any drugs, and it too was negative. Even his serum electrolytes were normal. Since he arrived at the ED some fourteen hours before, he had not had another similar spell, so he was in no predictable, imminent danger for which he would need to be hospitalized. As for admitting him to run more tests, the critical tests that we would have performed were already done.

"Hey Trina. I've been reading the ED notes on this kid," I said. "I'm a little confused about something. Why's he coming in?"

Trina looked at me with disgust. "*That's* a good question," she said. "I have no idea why they admitted him except to make a lot of work for us for a patient who *should* have been managed outpatient by the *headache clinic!*" It was only two-thirty in the afternoon and Trina was already mad about the work that lay ahead.

When I first came in to see him, I thought I was in for even more teenager trouble. He was resting, even though the television was on so loud I could scarcely hear myself when I spoke to him, and he indicated with some shrugging of his shoulders that now wasn't a great time to talk. I told him I'd drop by later, and he shrugged his understanding. I briefly thought about *not* returning, since virtually all of the information I needed to present him the following morning was in the chart, but decided that, in the interests of my education, I would come back later on.

A couple hours later I came back, and Clark seemed a changed young man. We talked for forty-five minutes, and I got a feel for what was really going on in this kid's life. It wasn't a great life. He was living in a group home because he had been essentially kicked out of his house by his mother because they had been fighting with each other too much. He was sexually and physically abused by his father, which had been the cause of several psychiatric admissions to Children's. He ended up back at the group home, in fact, because his mother wanted him admitted again; as she drove him toward the hospital, he realized what she was doing, and bolted from the car, running away to a friend's house. That took place last week.

Clark's one wish was to get out of the group home, and suddenly I felt like there was something I could do for one of the patients beyond observe their condition. He was going to be 18 in five months, anyway, and since his tox screen was negative it hardly sounded like a crazy request. Where he was going to live was not something he had a plan for, but I figured that I would at least check out whether or not moving out was feasible. I put in a message to Social Work to call me or drop by and see him.

Monday, January 28

Janice Levels is one of the more interesting cases I've come across so far. From a "purely" medical standpoint, there's nothing interesting about her at all, but still she is in the hospital and will likely be here for days. When we took call the other night I got a call from Trina, who asked me to come over to the Pavilion to talk to the mother and get the story. Trina seemed irritated at the time, and what I realized later was that she initially *tried* to get the story from the mom but simply couldn't keep her on track, and she had to take her leave to work up the five other patients that had been admitted thus far.

The Levels family seemed like a very nice, happy family at first — they are African-American, and probably from the inner-city. Some families can be hostile or suspicious of residents, and especially of medical students, but both mom and daughter seemed genuinely pleased that so many doctors had dropped by to see them (in addition to Trina, the senior resident and the Neurology team had come to the room to evaluate her). So, I asked, what brought her in here?

As the story progressed, I began to feel a little uneasy, for, as mom kept talking, I began to realize that she reminded me of the manics I worked with during psychiatry. She simply *never* stopped talking, even when I tried as politely as possible to interrupt, and often she did not make a whole lot of sense. It was nearly impossible to figure out what was going on. About all I learned after an hour was that Janice began to feel pain in her legs last week, and gradually lost function in her legs; she was finally admitted when she could no longer walk. This appeared to bear no relation to any kind of trauma or precipitating illness. I performed an exam on her and her reflexes were stone-cold normal, with normal-looking legs. I didn't see a hint of trauma, or anything else that looked suspicious.

"Have the Neurology doctors told you what they suspect?" I asked.

"Oh yes! Yes, yes, yes!" She said. "Those doctors, I tell you, they are so *smart*, I am so glad that we have Children's Hospital here with all these smart people. Did you know that there were *three* of them, all came at the same time? They came with all of these tools for an examination. I was amazed at what they did! They had this strange-looking tool to do the thing that you did with that hammer…"

"And what did they tell you?"

"There was one tall, white man, I think he was the one in charge, then there was another who seemed, I don't know, Indian maybe. You know, not Indian, like from America, but from India…"

"And, um, *what* did they tell you?"

"Oh! I wrote it down here. Wait a minute, I put it in my purse…yes, here it is! They called it 'Pain Amplification

Syndrome.' That's it. Do you know how quickly they can fix it?"

I had never heard of Pain Amplification Syndrome. "Well, I'll talk with the Neurology team and see if we can get a plan together, then I'll let you know about it as soon as I know something. Okay?"

I caught up with Trina later. "Well, weren't *they* a lot of fun?" she asked.

"*What* is Pain Amplification Syndrome?" I asked back.

"It means that kid's taking up a hospital bed for someone who's *really* sick while we babysit her until the psych unit has a bed available," she said. "The only thing's wrong with that kid is her mother is crazy, and *we* have to take care of her in the meantime."

"When will a psych bed open up?" I asked, although I knew from my experience in the Child Psych ward in October that kids can wait up to a week, even 10 days for a psych bed. Amazingly, during those days, they typically get little if any psychiatric help: The psych service is just spread too thin.

Trina rolled her eyes. "Well, I'd put it this way. Don't hold your breath."

That was a few days ago. Since then, any *mention* of the Levels family is enough to turn Trina's skin a lovely shade of red. "It's not fair," she's said on more than one occasion. "It's not fair to *us* to have to take care of some kid who's got nothing wrong with her, and it's not fair to some other kid sitting in the emergency overflow area because all the hospital beds are taken. She needs to go home so that we can take care of kids who are *really* sick!"

Thursday, February 1

Jesus, bless my senior-resident-for-a-day.

Actually, don't bless him. But you can deliver him a payback good deed at some point for letting me out of my last call tonight. About 3:30, after I finished up my "observed" history and physical exam, I called the new resident on call, Alex, and asked her what I should do for the night. She said talk to the senior, so I called up Sam, the new guy on the block replacing Art and Scott of beloved memory, and asked him what to do. I was not expecting a favorable reply, as only a three-hour exposure to Sam had not given me the best impression.

He said, "As far as I'm concerned, you guys finished your work when the last team left, so if you *want* to take call tonight, then you're certainly welcome to, but if your resident doesn't have any objections, then feel free to get out of here and get as much free time as you can." Sam, who had rounded with us earlier that morning, and who appeared to be painfully thorough, had not led me to believe that he would make such a statement.

It's pretty awful for me, a student toying with the idea of doing pediatrics for residency, to so openly admit to not wanting to take call, especially my last one. But to take call the day after Switch Day, when the teams have changed and the people you've been getting to know for an entire month are gone, almost seems pointless. I suppose that there is learning to be done by picking up patients, but mostly my thoughts were of coming home and hanging out with Miriam, whom I hadn't seen the entire month.

Sunday, February 11

I have to go in to the Newborn Nursery at the University in three hours, and although I had a good experience when I went last Wednesday night, I am not much looking forward to going. I don't feel like I've had much time to come up for air since I started peds—I've had only two consecutive days off in five weeks—and with the test looming just around the corner, I'm worried I won't have enough gas in my can to get me through to the end. Of course, this is only a small sampling of what residents go through for three to five consecutive *years*, and they get much less sleep than I do. So either I shouldn't complain or residents should be prepared to go to war. Or both.

It's been a long week, and not all of it good. I assumed that as soon as I began my outpatient experience I'd be on Easy

Street. I had even heard rumors that I'd be out of the office after only three or four hours each day, as many classmates who worked outpatient in January said that they worked twenty-hour weeks. I figured I'd take advantage of the extra time and catch up on some writing, as well as get some serious study time in for this allegedly hellacious shelf exam in three weeks.

People speak of this shelf exam with *fear*. I was talking to a peds-psych resident while I was on my psychiatry rotation, telling her how hard I found the psych shelf exam to be. "Oh, that's nothing," she said. "Just *wait* until you take the peds exam. It was the hardest test I've ever taken in my life, and that includes the MCAT and the Boards."

For my outptatient experience, I had come on board with a guy who does standard nine-to-five hours. All things considered, it could have been worse; one of my classmates that I ran into at Grand Rounds on Tuesday morning works from 8 a.m. to 6 p.m. Monday through Friday, *and* has to work Saturday morning as well. Not only does he have to worry about having less time to study for the shelf exam, he's raising two kids as well.

Hours aside, the week didn't start off well. I arrived at the doctor's office — a group practice of about seven or eight physicians who have a good chunk of one of the floors of a medical office building — and introduced myself to the administrators and nurses. My preceptor, Aaron Blumstein, had not yet arrived, so I sat down in one of the chairs and opened up my review book in pediatrics. As I opened up the book, I saw a man, about forty years old, get escorted into one of the rooms that I'd been told were used by Dr. Blumstein. I wondered why he was seeing an adult. Then I thought about the name of the practice, *Suburban Family Physicians*, and got worried.

"Um, excuse me," I said to the nurse after she escorted the man into the exam room. "Is that man you just brought in one of Doctor Blumstein's patients?"

"Yes, he is," she said.

"Oh. Um, is he a *family* doc, by any chance?"

"Yes, he is," she said.

Great, I thought. I'm here to do pediatrics in an office setting, and here I've gotten assigned to an outpatient preceptor who is a family physician. Based on my experience with the Mittleschmertz clan back in September, I was afraid that I'd be seeing more adult & geriatric patients than kids. This was fine when I was working with the Mittleschmertzes, since that rotation was Family Medicine. But now, for this month, I wanted to see only kids, especially since I would be seeing plenty of adults during my outpatient medicine month coming up in either March or April.

Blumstein arrived about five minutes later, around ten past nine. The patients are scheduled for Dr. Blumstein starting at nine. Like so many doctors I've seen, Blumstein showed up late, and continued to run later and later as the day wore on, making patients wait longer and longer to see him. I've never been able to understand why doctors can't seem to figure out approximately how long it will take to see a patient and take care of their administrative tasks. It's like, *what — you don't know that your work day begins at nine?* Dr. B stands about five-five, and except for the height difference, I could almost look like a son of his: He's dark-haired with a salt-and-pepper beard, wearing glasses, has the mid-forties soft-in-the-middle belly. In short, he looks like the stereotypical Jewish doc. He saw me, came over and introduced himself.

"Hi, Aaron Blumstein. You must be the med student. Third or fourth year?"

"Third," I said. "I was wondering, are you a family doc?"

Silence for a second, and he eyeballs me. Trying to figure out if I've just insulted him or not, which I hadn't. He must have interpreted it that way, though, judging by the response. "I'm boarded in pediatrics and internal medicine, if that's what you're asking," he said. Meaning that he thought I was inquiring what kind of training he got. In the pecking order of physicians, a family physician is on one of the lowest rungs, whereas a med-peds doc is higher, since there are fewer med-peds programs, and the competition to get into such programs is more fierce. He thought I was trying to size him up.

"No, that's not what I meant," I said. Off to a great start and

I haven't even seen a patient. "I don't know if you're aware, but I'm doing my pediatrics clerkship, not family medicine or internal medicine. I just wanted to make sure that there wasn't some kind of mix-up."

"Oh. Well, I see kids, you know. Why, let's just look at the schedule for the day and see how many kids we've got." He goes over to the schedule, and starts moving his pen down the list. "Hmm. No, he's not. Hmmm. Mmmm. Okay. Well, today's not such a good day. We've got one kid coming in at four-thirty. But I do see kids regularly in my practice."

Wonderful. "Well, if you don't mind, I'm just going to call up Jeanne and double-check things with her to see if everything's in order."

"Sure, that's no problem. Phone's there. Nine to get out."

Call up the course secretary Jeanne and I can tell right away that she doesn't want to deal with this. "No, Steven, I'm sure you're going to see kids with this doctor. It will be fine," she said. "We've been working with him for some time now." Click.

It took me the better part of the morning to figure it out, but eventually I realized what was going on. She didn't assign me to a full-time kid doc because she didn't *have* one. There simply weren't enough pediatricians to go around. Or rather, there weren't enough pediatricians who were volunteering to take on medical students for a month or two.

Why there was such a paucity of volunteers in a city the size of Cincinnati is less clear, but I've got a couple of guesses. First is simply the financial aspect: Having a med student slows you down. If you volunteer to take on a med student for a month, it could easily reduce your ability to see, say, twenty percent of your patients. Obviously patients schedule appointments months in advance, so it's not like the docs will just call up patients and say, 'Sorry, but I've got a med student this month, and it's slowing me down. Don't come in today,' but they will likely take less patients that call in the morning looking for an appointment. At the end of the month, you will have generated less revenue for your business by taking on the burden of a student, pure and simple. And your compensation from the medical school is either minimal or nonexistent.

Another reason is that many docs simply don't *want* to teach, period. Third year students are profoundly ignorant, and while the learning curve is pretty steep—I feel considerably more competent than I did on my first day of surgery in July— to teach well you have to take time and be patient. Many docs are talented at being docs but less talented at being teachers— they know how to *be* a physician but don't know as well how to *explain* to someone else what's required to become one. This has been one of the biggest frustrations for me thus far.

A last reason is simply that the University may not have a great relationship with many of the pediatricians, and some people that have formerly been involved in student education may have decided not to participate anymore. This could easily happen if a doc had a student who managed to say or do something outrageously stupid to a patient. That's not too hard to envision. Plus the course directors, or the medical school personnel, could have said something that may have piqued a doc, and they decided a med student wasn't worth the grief. I don't know how much this last factor contributes to the problem but it seems distinctly possible.

As a consequence, I was standing there, holding the receiver in my hand, figuring out what on earth I was going to do that day with only *one* kid to see, and at that a kid that wasn't coming in for another seven hours. During this time Blumstein was seeing his patient, and when he came out he said, "What's up?"

"Nothing's afoot," I said. "I'm afraid you're stuck with me for the next month."

"*Month*? You're going to be here that long?" "I'm afraid so, if that's going to be okay by you."

Pause. "Yeah, it's no sweat. I'm used to having students. You guys keep me on my toes." He was beginning to sound like he was warming up, and at least we'd have some rapport together.

• • • • • • • •

As the week marched on, Blumstein did indeed warm up, and by the end of the week he was telling me how it's a pity that I want to go into research because I'd be such a good clinician. This certainly made me feel pretty good. Maybe I'll manage to even get a decent evaluation from him, I thought greedily.

Sometimes I came to feel a little uncomfortable around him. It wasn't his clinical skills, which as far as I was able to tell, are up to snuff. Rather, he's a very sociable doctor — maybe *too* sociable. He likes to chat with his patients, and he likes to chat with his patients about *himself.* By the end of the first week, I learned that he's coaching a basketball team and has to go buy a trophy for the kids, that his kids go to private day school, and that he managed to kill three out of four goldfish recently when cleaning their tank. All of this I learned by listening to the casual conversation with his patients.

Maybe some of them are personal friends, and maybe others don't mind the down-home and very informal approach he takes. I'd have less discomfort if he talked with his patients about *their* lives as much as his own.

I was also amazed at some of the hum-dingers he managed to deliver when dealing with patients. The best one was when I had just come in to see a 17 year-old young woman who had come in for some vague muscle pain. She was a nice kid. She and I talked for about ten, maybe fifteen minutes before I went to get Blumstein, and one of the things we talked about at the end was her parents' divorce and the impact its had on her. Obviously, this was a one-time meeting between us with a limited amount of time, so I was not going to probe too deeply, but even in that short time of a few minutes I was able to gather that she was upset about her 38 year-old father, who had recently taken to dating a 23 year-old college co-ed. "I mean, I think it's weird that she's closer in age to *me* than she is to *him*," she told me.

Blumstein came in and he immediately asked about how she was taking the divorce. It was pretty clear that she felt comfortable talking to him and spoke bluntly about her issues.

"She's twenty-three?" Blumstein asked. "Man, that's kind

of slimy, isn't it? It reminds me of my neighbors. Whoa! That's one *bad* divorce that went down. Before they sold the house *he* was living in the basement and *she* was living in the rest of the house, and they had the two parts locked off from one another so they didn't have to see each other. Then the wife, she starts calling everybody up on the street, and tells them that he was having an affair, that's why she's leaving him. Like, did I need to know that? It's not my business, you know?"

Tuesday, February 13

One of the requirements of the pediatric clerkship—you've understood that there are many requirements for this clerkship by now, I hope—is to spend two nights at the Newborn Nursery and Newborn Intensive Care Unit at University Hospital. The Nursery and NICU are staffed by pediatric docs, but because the Labor & Delivery ward is housed at the University Hospital, not Children's, the pediatric residents work in this corner of the University even though it's not their home turf. I came in last night at five, after a full day with Dr. Blumstein, and hooked up with my intern, a nearly-albino woman named Shelley who had done medical school in Illinois. This came out after we discussed that I would be going from the office, to call at the NICU, and back to the office the following day. "Jeez," she said. "When I was in Illinois, we were *never* on call. For *any* of our clerkships."

The Nursery and NICU is located on the 3rd floor in the "Pavilion" portion of the hospital. Like most major university medical centers (especially those east of the Mississippi), University Hospital is an amalgam of several different buildings built over the decades, all interconnected through tunnels and bridges, so that the whole is a sprawling, teeming mess of concrete and steel. The oldest buildings on the campus date back 100 years, while the Pavilion, the newest structure, was built in the past twenty. The Nursery and NICU is one giant room, something of a dimly lit cavern, occupying both the third and fourth floors.

Nursery children (i.e. those that are healthy and require no special interventions such as respirators or feeding tubes) are on one side of the room, while the NICU children (who consist mostly of preemies) are in three smaller pods on the other side, with about six children per pod. The dim lights, soft music, and high ceiling is designed to be newborn-friendly, and consequently *my* first impulse when I entered it was to look for the nearest blanket so I could cuddle up and take a nap.

The major teaching objective during these two overnight stays is to learn to perform a cursory newborn examination and write a brief note about it. Thus, when any new children are delivered in Labor & Delivery, the pediatric team is paged, and we come to evaluate the child at the time of delivery, then bring baby back to the nursery for a more complete evaluation, including a blood draw to assess sugar levels and screen for a few rare but disastrous diseases which can be rendered harmless if caught at birth, such as PKU, or phenylketonuria. After I got a brief orientation to the Nursery, Shelley and I went over to one of the healthy kiddos so that she could teach me a basic newborn exam.

If you haven't had the pleasure of watching them up close, newborns are an awesome display of the magic of human development, especially neural development. Think of how long it takes you as an adult to learn a foreign language; if you have talent, with concerted effort, you can master the basics in a few months, but you will *never* be able to negotiate fully the intricacies of grammar and syntax, and you'll always sound like an outsider. In just about five years, by contrast, kids not only fully master a language's grammar and basic vocabulary, but do it starting from nothing at all, and do it while they simultaneously teach their bodies to become fully coordinated!

If you're the kind of person that thinks that's an awesome display of the magic of evolution, then watching a newborn for a concentrated period of time is a special reward. A baby's neural circuitry is wired differently than an adult's, and one method of checking the development of that circuitry is to observe their reflexes. Everyone knows about the famous "patellar tap" reflex, where your leg will raise when tapped just below your kneecap. Newborns have such wild reflexes as the crossed-extensor, where a little rub on the sole of a left foot, with the left leg held in a specific way, will cause the *right* leg at first to pull up to the body, then kick out. They have a "Moro" reflex where, when startled, they shake both of their arms, a bit like how body builders flex their upper muscles. And by the age of two months, as the forebrain develops and gains more direct control over the body, these reflexes disappear.

These were among the items I was reviewing with Shelley. After we performed a dry run exam on a baby who had come into the nursery several hours earlier, she said, "Well, you'll be ready now when one comes in overnight and you'll be able to do one by yourself. Better get some sleep, because it could be a long night."

I tried to do some reading and drifted off around midnight. At about 2:30 the pager went off, and in the darkness I made out the letter "A" and immediately awoke, hearing everyone hastily scramble from their call rooms. An "A" code meant there was a newborn emergency and the pediatric team was needed immediately. This was usually called when a premature infant was delivered. In this case, the "A" code was in the ER, so everyone hit the stairs at breakneck pace. By the time we got down there, the ER docs were waving their arms. "Sorry guys, false alarm," one said. "This lady came in. She delivered her baby at home, and we didn't know what to expect, but they're both fine. You can take your time."

Mom had apparently felt a pressure in her pelvis, like her bladder was full. "I just went to the bathroom, you know? Then I feel like I'm having a big bowel movement and I realize I'm having the baby. I called my husband, and he called 9-1-1, and by the time he came back I had delivered her. I delivered the placenta a minute later, and the EMTs came a few minutes after that."

We took the baby up to the nursery, where I performed the exam I had been taught a few hours earlier, looking at the cheat-sheet that was supplied for the interns and medical students alike. We went back to bed just shy of four, and a half-hour later the pager went off again, this time noting it was a "B" code, which meant a routine birth, and we could take our time in going to the delivery room. The four of us—a second resident assigned to the NICU, a fourth-year student working with her, Shelley, and me—headed off to the delivery room, sauntering our way there.

Once we got there, though, it was apparent that something wasn't right. One of the OB nurses was escorting everyone but the husband out of the room. When we got to the baby, a little African-American boy, he was clearly blue and his breathing was labored. "What's going on?" the second resident, Nancy, had asked in irritation as she looked the child over. "We were called as a Code B!"

"I think things were fine until after the delivery," one of the nurses said. "Then he just seemed not to have a lot of energy. His Apgars were five and five." Apgars are immediate assessments of the baby's health at the first and fifth minute of life; an Apgar of eight or above (ten is the highest score) means the baby is fine; an Apgar of three means the baby needs immediate resuscitation. Five was not a good score.

Immediately Shelley, Nancy, and the fourth-year set their hands on the child, one listening to the baby's heart and lungs, the other two mostly rubbing him briskly to invigorate him. "What the hell's wrong with this baby," Nancy hissed. She then looked directly at me. "Go talk to the mom, and find out something, *anything*."

I had no idea what to say, and I had even less of an idea of what to do. Springing into action is one matter; going when you have absolutely no clue what action to take was another. What information did Nancy need? What could cause this kind of a presentation in a kid? I had to know this stuff in order to ask the right questions, but the problem was that I didn't know it. Maybe, if given a few minutes, I could slowly figure out the answer, but by the time I reached mom the only thing I could produce was sweat.

"Um, hi," I said as a warm-up. "Uh, we need to know some information. Have there been any complications during the pregnancy?" She shook her head no. Dad, by this time, had moved over by the baby, rocking back and forth on the balls of his feet and asking the Lord to please not take his baby away.

"Um, is this your first child?" I continued. She indicated it was her second, and told me that there were no problems with the first. I paused, not knowing what next to ask. At that point, Shelley had made her way over to the bed, seeing that I was obviously out of my range of skill, and she quickly made her way through a brief battery of questions, wanting to know if she had been tested for CMV, HIV, Rubella, what her blood type was, the father's blood type, and if she had any recent infections. Each question she asked, I thought, *Shit! That's what I should have asked!* By the time we finished these questions, the baby was beginning to breath with more energy, and Nancy explained that we were going to need to take him to the NICU. With that, the team whisked him away, and I trailed behind, feeling stupid, and partly responsible for nearly having killed a kid.

As we walked back Shelley looked over her shoulder at me and shook her head. "We'll talk later," she whispered. After the NICU nurses had been mobilized, Shelley, whose responsibilities like mine lay in the Nursery, came over to me and we sat in the nursery in the comfortable rocking chairs near the kids. I still had cold sweat pouring down my head; my glasses were half-fogged from the moisture and my scrubs were soaked through from the waist up. It was the first time since I began medical school where I very nearly cried. *I almost killed a kid*, I kept thinking.

"Listen, you shouldn't have been thrown into that. I don't know what Nancy was thinking."

"Should I have known what to ask?"

"No. You weren't ready. It's your first night, for Christ's sake. I should have stepped in to take over, but that kid didn't look good, and I just focused on him. When I realized what was happening I came over."

"Jesus, Shelley, I didn't know what to do."

"Listen, don't sweat it. You'll get a feel for this as we go along."

The baby turned out to do just fine, and by the time we began morning rounds a few hours later he had already been moved into the regular newborn nursery. Rounds were led by Dr. Ballard, one of the most famous doctors in Cincinnati. Dr. Ballard is known for the "Ballard exam," which provides an estimate of the child's gestational age based on the child's appearance, flexibility, and strength. It felt a little odd to present to Dr. Ballard the "Ballard score" and call it such, although she's heard it so many times by now that she's probably adjusted to it.

Rounds consisted of checking on every non-NICU newborn in the hospital. We also performed a few frenulotomies—a frenulum is that little bit of tissue in the midline on the underside of your tongue, and some babies have a little too much tissue, making their tongue less mobile, so a frenulotomy cuts just enough of it to allow full tongue mobility. By the late morning, when we finished rounds at 11:30, the memory of the near-disaster we had the night before didn't carry the emotional edge it had that morning.

I think one reason it was so scary was that it marked in many ways the first time I wasn't just *observing* a medical situation, but was actively part of the management of it. Oh, sure, I have written lots of notes, and sometimes on psychiatry I've even played a major part in a patient's care. But I was never critical to what happened, I was never *needed* for a patient's well-being. Most of what we do consists of watching and simulating while others critique us. Suddenly, last night, I was moved directly into a much more active role. It gave me a taste for what it feels like when you actually have to *make* the decisions, and it was pretty damn scary.

Thursday, February 15

We pause from this narrative on pediatrics to bring you words from the department of general surgery and one of our most popular subjects, Joshua Lipschitz. Today's stories come courtesy of classmate Rod Stefano, who is pondering applying for surgical residencies. We were trading Lipschitz stories, and Rod, who had actually been assigned to work with Lipschitz on several occasions, confirmed that Lipschitz in fact does not talk to medical students under normal circumstances.

"Yeah, one time he even explained to us why he doesn't," he said. "He said, 'Yelling at a medical student is like yelling at a retarded person. It doesn't get you anywhere.'"

Every once in a blue moon, though, Rod says, a medical student can impress the old man. This one involves a classmate named Chris. "One day there was this appendectomy going on, and Chris was the student assigned to the case. Lipschitz came in late, after the resident had already begun to cut the patient. That was fine, but the resident was totally in the wrong place, dissecting out some plane of anatomy that wasn't headed toward the appendix. Lipschitz comes in, sees what's going on, and says, 'Where the *fuck* are you? What the *fuck* are you doing?'

"Chris steps in and says, 'Oh, I'm sorry, Doctor Lipschitz, I was just asking him if he'd show me some of the anatomy before you came.' Lipschitz looked at him and said, 'That's nice, trying to cover for him. I guess you're a team player. I like that.' It's possible that Chris got Honors in surgery for that single comment."

Friday, February 16

Blumstein says to me today: "Your wife working on Monday?" President's Day Weekend is upon us.

"No, she's not."

"Oh. Well, why don't you take the day off and go do something with her."

"Okay, but I'll only do it to make *her* happy."

It reminds me of a conversation I had with one of the surgery residents. We were talking about how much work you did at the hospital as a student and when was it time to leave. The resident was of the opinion that you didn't *ask* to leave early, but if it was offered, you should turn and say 'you sure? I can stay and help' as you are retreating away from whomever told you to take off. If that person says *no, get out of here*, you should move with the approximate speed, and in the cartoon fashion manner, of the Road Runner.

• • • • • • • •

My shtick with kids has gotten pretty good, and I think I can get most of them to ease up while I examine them. For instance, I have a routine to relax the kids in the 4-to-10 year age range when I examine their eyes. "Follow my finger," I tell them. Or the otoscope, or the reflex hammer, whatever I'm holding. I move my hand slowly like I'm drawing a large "H" in front of them, followed by an "X", to assess the competency of the nerves and muscles responsible for eyeball movement. At the end, I either wrap my hand behind their head or move it very quickly in a zig-zag. The kids usually smile or laugh, the parents think I'm cute, I feel good about my social skills. It's all very win-win for everyone.

Still, you can't win everyone over. Two days ago I'm examining a five year-old for a sore throat. I do my eye-test number and watch the kid not react very much — not that she found it dumb, but just didn't seem to find it much of anything, and I couldn't write it off to her being a sick kiddo, since she was doing fairly well. Mom was amused and made some pleasant noises, but I got worried. How was the rest of the exam going to go?

I got my answer soon enough. I moved through my exam. Listened to her heart, lungs, belly. Looked in her ears. Tried to look in her mouth but she just couldn't manage to get her tongue out of the way, so I knew I'd have to go back later and get a tongue depressor to get a good look at her throat. Felt her abdomen, which I thought was going to cause screaming, but she was perfect. Then I go to get my tongue depressor, and said, "Now I just want to get a better look inside your mouth. Can you say, 'Ahh'?"

She opened up, I put my tongue depressor right at the tip of her tongue, and all hell broke loose. A SCREAMING kid is now sitting on the table. It so surprised me I nearly fell over; it so surprised mom, who had been sitting in a chair a few feet away, that she apparently teleported to the exam table, instantaneously, to comfort her. Sobbing now, with kid-snot coming out of her nose. *Jeez!* — I think. *What'd I do?*

"I'm so sorry," mom said. "I think it's from the last time when she came in for this infection..."

"And she got a strep test, am I right?" I asked. I was right. If you haven't had the pleasure, a strep test involves taking a q-tip and swabbing the back of one's throat on both sides. I have never had one administered on me but it appears deeply unpleasant. I've seen lots of people, kids included, tolerate needlesticks and shots, but I've now seen probably twenty or so strep tests and not one has been much-liked by the recipient.

In the meantime, I was worried about what everyone in the office *outside* the exam room was thinking. More specifically, I was worried that they were thinking something along these lines: *What the hell's that medical student doing to Dr. Blumstein's patients?* After I finished the exam, I told them that Dr. Blumstein will be in shortly to see them. I came out and saw the medical assistant raise her eyebrows at me. "It go all right in there?" she asked.

"I was doing all right until we got to the tongue depressor," I said. "Doctor Blumstein, I can't tell if the kid's got strep because I couldn't look in the back of her throat. I wasn't going to push the issue."

"And you were right to do it that way, Doctor Hatch. Let's go take a look."

He, too, couldn't get a good look without the tongue depressor, and when he reached for it, she screamed at roughly the pitch and decibel level of a DC-10. Good, it's not just me. He wrote her a scrip for antibiotics just as a precaution.

Monday, February 19

As time has gone on, and I've worked with a variety of preceptors, I've come to understand that what they do is a hard job, and *how* they do their job is dependent upon their personalities. I'm often critical of them when I first work with them, thinking, "well, *I* wouldn't do that!" or, "don't they know that's *wrong*?" when I see them handle a situation that obviously wasn't drawn up in the playbook. But then, as time goes by, I'll realize that they work in their own way, that there's no "right" way to deal with a patient (although there could be several "wrong" ways), and that I'm going to bring my own unique quirks to the job which some will find helpful while others will not.

Thus, I've adjusted to Dr. Blumstein's very sociable style. And I've realized that most of his patients rather like his chatty approach. One day, I came into the exam room of a fifty year-old (a nice pediatric specimen), and as I questioned him on various medical issues, he wanted to know about what exactly a medical student does. As we conversed, the topic turned to his relationship with Blumstein.

"How long have you been seeing him as a patient?" I asked.

"Oh, gosh, it's been a long time. About ten years, I figure," he replied.

"That's a long time," I said. "He was located somewhere else ten years ago. You followed him out here?"

"Yeah, it's good to stay with the same guy. He knows me and what's going on with me, you know? I trust him."

He then looked off in the distance for a second and chuckled. "Yeah, he *sure* is a talker."

Tuesday, February 20

Last Thursday night on the TV show *ER* there was a story line about a child who had come in with signs of meningitis, but also had a funky rash. Dr. Carter (Noah Wyle) walks into the room where the kid was being treated, looks at him, and says that maybe the kid's got measles. The other resident says no way, can't be measles, after all, the kid's vaccinated, right? Carter looks inside the kid's mouth for the classic measles sign of "Koplik's spots" and finds them just as the mother comes walking in. "Is this kid up to date on his immunizations?" asks Carter.

"We don't believe in immunizations for our children," mom responds. The doctors exchange knowing glances— knowing that mom is a dumbass, that is—and as the episode continues, mom says angrily to Carter that she's read the literature showing that immunizations aren't as safe as they claim to be and that they are linked to autism. Carter argues with her, but to no avail. Later in the show, the kiddo dies from encephalopathy caused by the measles, and Carter is left shaking his head in resigned disbelief.

After the episode, I was surging with energy. "You know, the producers of the show couldn't have handled that situation any better than they did," I said to Miriam, pointing my finger sharply at the TV. "There are these *nuts* out there who think that it's bad to get your kid immunized, and the show took an unambiguous stand on that kind of thinking. I'm glad that they wrote that kind of situation in to show how *crazy* these people are!" I prattled on for another few minutes, Miriam politely pretending to listen to my diatribe, before we both went to bed.

I wasn't done, though. The episode had me pumped. The next morning, as I was driving up to the office, I was having angry fantasies about what *I* would have said to that family had I been Carter. It took me four or five tries—about the length of the car ride—but I had my speech pretty well rehearsed by the end. It went like this:

I march down the corridor after the kid expires. I'm seething. I look the parents straight in the eye and keep walking. I pass by, and make some collegial remark to another doctor who has walked by. The mother is following me. She catches up to me and turns me around and says, "you're not going to say anything to me? You're not going to tell me that you're sorry that my son is dead?"

"I'm sorry that your kid is dead, but I am definitely not sorry for you," I respond. "He's dead because of you. You might as well have put a gun to his head and played Russian roulette, or sent him out to play on an interstate. As far as I'm concerned, someone should call the cops on you, because what you did was criminally negligent homicide. But there's one thing you should feel good about, mom. At least you know your son doesn't have autism."

You'll see where this is going in a second.

• • • • • • • •

By twelve-thirty this afternoon, I had managed to see two, yes, count 'em, *two* kids. I pulled Dr. Blumstein aside and asked him what the afternoon was going to be like in terms of seeing any *more* kids. He looked down the appointment printout and saw that he was booked solid until five o'clock with fifty-and-overs with one single exception, a ten year-old girl who was a follow-up for attention-deficit disorder.

Blumstein obviously felt bad for me and said, "You know, I was hoping that some of the other docs around here were going to be more willing to pull you aside when they had kids to see. Let's go check out their schedules and see what they've got cooking." And so we moved around the office, looking at the various printouts that each doctor had for their daily schedules.

"Oh, here's something," Blumstein said. "This kid is a new patient in for a one-month well-child checkup. Let's ask Doctor Pansaron if it's okay with her if you shadow her on this one. She may not since they are new patients, and it might be uncomfortable to have an extra person in the room. Maybe not, though."

"Well, listen, I don't want to make any waves with your colleagues," I said.

"She's your colleague, too. If she doesn't want to do it, she'll say so, no big deal."

Which was true, and Pansaron, a doc in her mid-forties, didn't mind. We went in to see this one-month old, a kid named Shlomi. When Blumstein and I saw the name on the printout we both looked at each other and agreed that the family must be either Jewish or Arab given the Semitic name. Instead, Dr. Pansaron and I walked in on two very young-looking hippie-types, probably in their early twenties. They had a pretty cute, bubbly baby (their first), and although they seemed young and weren't wearing my style of clothing, nothing seemed amiss.

At the outset, though, they made it clear that they were still in the "looking" phase for a doctor, and they had come to Pansaron because one of the midwives had recommended her due to her reputation of being able to work with patients who used "alternative medicine." Pansaron didn't react, and let the parents continue. "We're anti-immunization, and we need to know if you're willing to work with us knowing that fact," dad said. You could tell they had been rehearsing their lines just like I had been rehearsing mine. You could also tell that he wasn't rock-solid confident in himself, like a kid trying to tell his mother that he knows better than she does. And Pansaron could easily have been this guy's mother.

Pansaron paused, and then said, "Of course I wouldn't refuse someone from my practice for this. I'm open to patients who are interested in alternative methods. I think some of it is good and some of it is not good at all. Have you taken a look at the German Pharmacopeia?" They both shook their heads. "Well, it's a book like the PDR or the Merck Manual, but they've included everything ever published about alternative medications, everything known about them. It's a very good resource for people who are interested in alternative methods."

They nodded approvingly. Again, it was *dad* that seemed to be supplying most of the cues; mom didn't seem adamant about the idea so much as wanting to agree with her husband. "It's really great that you're aware of what's going on outside of western medicine," he said.

Oh, Lord, I thought. When will it be time to sing *kum-ba-ya*?

"But let me ask you a question," Pansaron said. "When you say that you're 'anti-vaccine,' does that mean that you don't want him to get *any* vaccinations?"

Dad looked a little puzzled, like vaccinations were supposed to be an open-and-shut case, and this conversation had suddenly taken an unexpected turn. "Well, um...which vaccinations do you *absolutely* recommend?"

"There are some that I really think he needs. Does he need the hepatitis B vaccine? Probably not, unless either of you have known hepatitis B. Does he need the polio vaccine? Again, probably not, since the odds of him getting it are so low since it's been eradicated from North America. But I *do* think that you need to seriously consider giving him the pertussis vaccine, since there have been small epidemics here in Cincinnati, especially in Finneytown, and a few children have died from it in the past few years. And I think it's quite wise to get the hemophilus influenza B vaccine."

A short discussion ensued as to why she thought those two vaccines were critical, and the major thrust of her argument was: *Do you want to risk your kid being dead?* Not that she phrased it this way, of course; she was as non-threatening as she could possibly be, never showing an ounce of hostility. She treated them as if they were rational adults, which they weren't, and she talked to them as if they had arrived at their decision after careful and well-informed research, which they hadn't. Of course, she had to approach them this way: Had they caught one whiff of condescension they wouldn't have returned, and possibly sought someone who shared their beliefs, such as a homeopath or a chiropractor—in short, a quack.

We went through the exam and they left saying they would think about what she had told them and whether they would decide to continue on with her. I never spoke during the entire session as this was my first time with Pansaron, and I wasn't going to speak unless she asked me if I had anything to say, but I was dying to know *why* they were opposed to immunizations. What particular form of nonsense had driven them to take this stand?

As they left, Pansaron looked at me and said, "Well, *that* wasn't exactly a routine well-child check, now was it?"

"It was perfect," I responded. "How often does that happen to you?"

"Oh, about two or three times a year, and that's pretty much my policy. I feel like it's their decision, and who am I to impose my will on them? Is it stupid, yes, but that's not for me to decide. It's like some doctors who refuse to take Jehovah's Witnesses, saying that they can't take care of their kids if they can't transfuse them when they get really sick. I don't know, but that seems wrong to me—you shouldn't refuse to treat someone just because they have views about treatment that you don't share."

"Fair enough, but don't you feel like you could be putting other patients in your practice at risk when you have them come walking through your door?"

"You mean by having them in the same waiting room? No, I'm not too worried about that. It would take more than that kind of casual contact to spread these bugs."

"What about MMR?" I asked, referring to the Measles-Mumps-Rubella vaccine, which I was astonished that she left off her must-vaccinate list. "You don't think that that's one he needs?"

"Oh, he won't need that until he's fifteen months old."

"So you're saying: Fight that battle another day?"

"Exactly. Fight that battle another day. I didn't want to push too hard. They're going to have problems down the road as it is. If they want to get their kid into a daycare center or into public school, they're going to discover that he won't be able to get in unless he's immunized. It's going to be a bumpy ride in a couple of years if they aren't aware of that right now."

"And you didn't want to let them know about that?"

Pansaron raised her eyebrows at me and smiled. "Hey, let *them* walk into that trap. If they want him to go to school and they haven't immunized him properly, he's going to need to get upwards of sixteen or seventeen shots. It's not my problem. I don't want to involve myself in something more than I already have."

I thanked her, and just as I was about to leave to go back to Blumstein, she added, "You know, I used to work up in this small practice in a small town in Minnesota. There were a bunch of these families and it was some religion, I can't remember now what exact group. I think it might have been related to the Mennonites. Anyway, they refused vaccines for their kids. One summer, these kids went away to a campground together, and there was a measles outbreak among them. Two of them died. Mind you, this is out of only about *fifty* kids in the entire town. It was awful.

"Then, later in the summer, we used to see families late into the day. Around seven we'd close the office, and just before we'd close up, a family would come through the door and ask if they could see us. We'd say sure, and once everyone was gone they'd ask us if they could immunize their children. They were taking them in at that hour because they didn't want anybody else knowing that they were doing this. But this was happening almost every night—probably most of that community ended up getting immunizations, but they didn't let each other know about it because they were afraid of being shunned."

Wednesday, February 21

I walk into one of the exam rooms and see a guy who's about twenty. He's wearing a Yankees ballcap with the bill curved sharply toward the floor. These are the patients that always worry me when I walk into the room: Male, adolescent or post-adolescent. Guys who are *very* hard to reach, at least for me.

He's not, though, and it's immediately apparent that it will be an enjoyable office visit: He's got a wisecracking look on his face like this is playtime.

"Hey, I'm Doctor Hatch. I'm a student doctor working with Doctor Blumstein today, he'll be in in a little bit, but I'm here to check you out in the meantime. So, what brings you in today?"

"My mom's been nagging at me to see the doctor because my throat's been sore. I need you to tell me that I'm sick so that you can get her off my back."

"No problem. Open wide," I say. I look in his mouth; he's a Strepper, clear as day. "Yep, you're sick."

That was easy.

Saturday, February 24

Yesterday, my last with Dr. Blumstein, was finally an all-pediatric day at the office. I saw about ten patients, only one of whom was over the age of 20. Not a bad way to end things at the Family Practice office. I suppose I should feel okay that I'm a little prepped for the medicine rotation. Which, incidentally, is going to be inpatient on the first month and outpatient the second month, like it was this time. I prefer that schedule since it gives me time to study over the second month and relax a little bit. In addition, I'll be back at the VA during my inpatient month, a place for which I've developed a great fondness.

But back to pediatrics. We had a kid come in at the very end of the day, when I was quite eager to get the hell out of there. It was pushing six and, as usual for Dr. Blumstein, we were running somewhere between one and two hours behind. This kid, a ten year-old, has a disorder called "central ataxia," which means that she's constantly writhing, and she's not capable of performing accurate, fluid movements with her limbs. I had seen her briefly last week for abdominal pain and vomiting; a week had passed and she wasn't getting much better.

Since she was the last patient of the day, Blumstein and I teamed up instead of our usual arrangement in which I went first and presented to him. We came in and she was hanging out on the exam table. As we're talking to mom about her symptoms, one thing that does get mentioned is her reticence to speak. I knew from the week before that she spoke, but was just a quiet kid. Blumstein either didn't remember speaking to her or may have just interacted verbally with mom on the last visit, and he asked her some questions to cover his bases. He asked her her age, where she went to school, her name, all of which she politely answered.

"So she's a quiet kid. You know, it reminds me of this joke," Blumstein said. "This kid, he's five years old, and he never speaks. Mom is beside herself. She doesn't know what to do. She's taken him to a dozen specialists and they've run dozens of tests, and nobody seems to know what's wrong.

"Then, one morning, the boy is having breakfast, and he turns to her and says, 'Mom, these eggs are cold. I'd like you to heat them up, please.'

"Mom looks at him and she's amazed. 'My God,' she says. 'All these years and now you're finally speaking! And in complete sentences!'

"The boy looks back at her and says, 'Well, the service has been pretty good up until now.'"

The girl and her mother gave blank stares at the joke, but Blumstein looked at the girl with this huge grin and grabbed her stomach playfully, saying, "I'm just fooling with you!" And while she didn't get the punch line, she clearly understood Blumstein's playful nature, because her face lit up with the brightest smile I have seen this entire month.

If I go into pediatrics, one of the top three reasons will be the memory of that kid's face.

Tuesday, February 27

The finish line is in sight, and I am ending my pediatrics rotation at an appropriately-named facility: Mercy. There are several Catholic-based Mercy hospitals around the city, and my requirement for the final week is to work in the Newborn Nursery at Mercy Anderson with one of the neonatology fellows.

"Mercy" is an appropriate name because the fellow asked me a few questions after I arrived for this final segment of the pediatrics course, and in the course of answering them I indicated that my final exam was this Friday. "I hear it's hard," said the fellow, who did medical school and residency somewhere in Scandanavia and came here for the fellowship.

"So I've been told on one or two occasions," I said.

"Well, listen. Why don't we do this: Let's get in a couple of good teaching hours in the morning, and I'll get you out before eleven each morning, and we'll let you have Thursday to study. How's that sound?"

How's *that* sound? Like *mercy*.

The neonate wing of Mercy Anderson is a tiny little place, with spots for maybe a half-dozen healthy babies and a couple of incubators for the preemies. It's certainly not as big as the enormous wing seen at the University. Mercy Anderson is the quintessential suburban hospital: Lots of plush carpeting everywhere, beautiful landscaping, tons of parking space and no parking garages.

None of this was on my mind as I came into the parking lot at five till eight this morning. The only thing on my mind was: Get in, get out, come home and STUDY! Or else my butt is gonna get kicked something fierce.

I can't recall a thing that I was taught during the two hours that passed this morning, and it's pretty clear my resident saw that, despite my natural curiosity and usual desire to learn, I was going to be a lost cause. At ten, he said, "Do you know what you want to go into?"

"I'm not sure yet."

"Are you thinking about pediatrics?"

"I am, and I really want to do well in this course."

"Let me guess: That means doing well on the test? That's fine. I'll see you tomorrow and I promise to keep it short. Now get out of here." Bless you, father.

NEXT STOP: DREADED TEST OF DOOM!

Friday, March 2

Out like a lamb.

It's hard to describe the kind of freedom I feel after I finish the final exam of a clerkship. I know that I have one entirely free weekend during which I have absolutely no responsibilities whatsoever, not to mention that I can exhale from all of the studying that I've been doing in the last forty-eight hours. Perhaps this isn't the most appropriate description, but the kind of feeling I get when I finish an exam is not unlike what crack addicts say about their excitement when they know they are going to score. It's a super-giddiness accompanying the feeling that nothing can touch you.

After the exam, Andrea and I headed over to the medical school and ran into practically everybody who had finished this-or-that course. The happiest people, of course, were those that walked away from surgery. You knew who they were by looking at the glow that surrounded them. My classmate Vikash was one of them, and Andrea and I roped him and Stuart Abbah into going to Cincinnati's best pizza place, Dewey's, for a celebratory lunch.

Shooting the breeze at lunch, Andrea, Vikash and I took it upon ourselves to scare the shit out of Stuart, who was starting his surgery rotation on Monday. It worked. By the end, we had Stuart visibly upset about what lay ahead for him. "I don't understand why someone doesn't let him have it!" he would say in reference to one of our stories about some horribly obnoxious remark made by Dr. Lipschitz. Or: "What would they do if someone came up to them, you know, after we've matched and everything, and just started screaming at them about how stupid they are?"

He was fairly animated, and I said, "Whoa, Stuart, it's not *that* bad. You'll make it through, no need to kill anybody." It's only two months, after all. But how the residents do it is beyond me.

Also at lunch: Vikash says, "Man, I am *so* happy to be done with surgery."

"Don't worry. That feeling will wash away in, oh, about one or two months," I said in reply.

"*This is how I picture how the medicine team should work. We're like a family. The attending is like Mom or Dad, the final authority, the last word, the person you don't necessarily want to share everything with, and sometimes the person who's going to spank you to keep you in line. The team leader is like the big brother or big sister. They're there to be helpful and supportive, and to pull you out of the messes that you'll get into. The interns are like the younger brothers and sisters, and the acting interns are like toddlers. Third years? Well, I like to think of them as the family pet.*"
— Chris Knight, MD, Medicine resident

<u>six</u>

<u>medicine</u>

Monday, March 5

All-day orientation. I had only a brief conversation with my team leader, a second-year resident named Chris Szymanowski (I have no idea how to pronounce his name yet), and explained that I'd be out of my orientation to the VA computer system around 4:30. "Dude, don't worry about it," he said. "We'll see you at seven-thirty tomorrow morning, dude." Okee-dokee.

Orientation was tedious, filled with the same information that we've heard many times before, including a review of expected professional conduct, the course grading system, the justification for the grading system, the weekly schedule, et cetera. The only amusing moment came when Ed Torrence, one of the younger attendings, said to us, when reviewing the weekly schedule, "I know what you *really* want to know. Okay, let me make a graph. This column is for the *days* we have conferences, this column is for the *locations* of the conferences, and this column indicates whether or not there is a *free lunch.*"

I'm over at the VA again working on Team Two. The team number has no special designation other than they take call and receive patients on such-and-such a day, which in our case will be Wednesday and every four days thereafter. I'm working with two Acting Interns (4th year students who are given the responsibilities of interns for one month) whose names I don't recognize, but Chris tells me that I'll be working most closely with a "true" intern, Jenny Wang. Tomorrow I'll hopefully have something more interesting to say about them than just their names.

Also noted—twice, in fact—during the morning session: When a code is called, what are the odds that the patient will walk away, alive and neurologically intact? That depends whether or not you watch *ER*, *Chicago Hope*, and *Rescue 911*, or instead you read the stats in the leading medical journals. If you follow the latter, then you know the odds are about one in one hundred that the patient will make it. In effect, a coded patient is a dead one.

On the TV shows, patients fare better. They have a 65 percent chance of full recovery.

Tuesday, March 6   pre-call

The cast and crew:

I'm assigned to Jenny Wang. She's in her intern year but she's not a medicine doc, instead moving on to the Dermatology residency when she finishes. She's from California and graduated from Michigan (woo woo). She wanted to go back home, but instead chose a specialty where she couldn't dictate her choices since it's such a highly competitive residency. Thus, she is here in Cincinnati. But she's outta here on the first bus after residency, so she told me today. The upside of having a derm resident is that I get someone very smart to work with; the downside is that she told me she doesn't much *want* to be doing medicine, since this is just a way-station for her. Her enthusiasm for the job is pretty low.

There are two acting interns, both fourth-year medical students, and both perfectly representative of the most common type of medical student in Cincinnati. Bob Struggins and Katrina Black are born-and-bred Cincinnatians. They went "away" to undergraduate (Bob to somewhere in Ohio, Katrina away to central Indiana), came straight back for medical school, got married to their respective high school sweethearts, and plan to stay in the area for residency and settle down, Bob in radiology, Katrina in family medicine. They seem nice enough, and I don't anticipate having anything other than pleasant, low-impact encounters with them for the rest of the month.

The other intern, Mina, is also from California and is not part of the medicine residency. She is completing a "preliminary" year in medicine before joining the Psych residency. Although she's an American, she was not able to attend an American medical school, and instead opted to do medical school in the Caribbean with the goal of returning to the States for residency. Apparently it took some trying, though: She applied to eleven programs the first time around and got rejected, then got a job working as a research assistant on Parkinson's patients at Duke (!), which seemed to do the trick in getting her in the next time around.

The chief of the team is Chris Szymanowski. Chris is from Philadelphia, where he went to school at Jefferson after an aborted career as an engineer and veterinary assistant. In fact, even in medicine he is a wayfarer, having started out in the psych residency, and then switched over to medicine. He seems to like the style of life that Bob and Katrina covet, since he's planning on staying around after he finishes residency.

I haven't had any interactions with Chris at all, except for this morning, when I realized that I had locked my white coat in my locker on the 9th floor but had forgotten to bring my key, which I had additionally forgotten to put on my keychain. So when I got to the hospital this morning, I realized that I didn't have an obvious way to get my coat, which was bad, nor could I get the stethoscope *in* my coat, which was worse. During rounds, I followed around without my jacket, feeling naked as a jaybird and stupid to boot, thinking that Chris has just got a *great* first impression of me. First day! Oy vay!

We had about twenty minutes between work rounds and attending rounds, so I went down to see Bridgette, the medical student coordinator, to see if she had an extra key. She did, and within minutes I had my white coat back on, had returned the key to her, and was on the elevator returning to the 6th floor, where the medicine teams base themselves. Chris picked up the elevator on the 3rd floor, came in, and looked at me. Was he aware that I didn't have my coat on earlier, or did he even care? I smiled lamely, hoping he would say something. He didn't. "Boy, it sure feels good to have my coat back," I said. "I felt exposed without it."

He returned my comment with a quizzical and somewhat amused look, which I read as *kid, what on earth are you talking about?* Oh, boy, I thought. One day and I'm off to a kicking start with my chief.

Saturday, March 10   pre-call

Whap.

Meaning: Whap — and a week goes by.

I've not had a chance to write down anything since Tuesday night. Wednesday was call, so that was obviously out, and on Thursday, when I came home from the hospital at six o'clock, I had intended to do some studying and some writing, but I ended up sleeping from the moment I got in until Friday morning. Yesterday I studied at the library after a lecture from five until nine, then Vikash and I went and got dinner. We came back home, had a couple of beers with Miriam, and then I conked out.

That brings us up to now, and I don't have any reason to believe that the remaining three weeks are going to be much easier. Fortunately, I have the entire day today off, so I can get somewhat caught up on writing and studying, and next weekend is something akin to a "golden weekend," a weekend with no call Friday, Saturday, or Sunday. Anyway, I expect that will be my free time to catch up with writing and everything else.

The quick news about my team is that I don't particularly *like* anyone on my team, but I don't particularly dislike anyone, either. We don't seem to work as a "team" so much as a bunch of people who round together and take call together. From what I've been able to see, the team members don't interact with each other outside of rounds, but instead follow their own patients individually.

Some of that has to do with their respective levels of experience. Bob and Katrina, the acting interns, are hustling just to keep up with following their own patients, and since they are very new to assuming full responsibility for a patient's hospital care, they're not going to be focusing on much outside of their own cases.

A story about Bob. He's a nice guy, but I'm also discovering with each passing day just how conservative he is, and frankly the more I learn the more frightening it gets. We were sitting around deciding about what to get for dinner for the team last night.* I said that I was partial to Indian food, but figured that Bob wasn't going to go for it, so I said I'd happily eat pizza but would eat anything else. Jenny and Katrina expressed similar sentiments. By the time Mina had come in, we had settled on the idea of burritos—not a native Caucasian dish, to be sure, but one sufficiently incorporated into American cuisine that we didn't think Bob would have a problem with it. He did, of course, puckering his lips and frowning at the mention of it.

"Bob, how can you not like burritos? They're pretty bland," Jenny said.

"Man, if it isn't meat or potatoes, I'm not very interested."

A story about Jenny. I've worked with Jenny for a week now and I've noticed something interesting. After we round, usually around 10 a.m., we head back to a resident work room and sit at the computers strewn about the room in order to type morning notes, order tests and meds, and check the daily labs. The computer system is remarkable, as any med student who works at any VA in the nation could tell you (since the system is nationwide). However, the system is only as good as the speed at which the work gets done: If the labs ain't finished, then they ain't no labs to be found on the computers.

On a daily basis, labs run behind at the VA, either because the laboratory is stretched too thin (likely) or because the workers are inept (possible). Thus, instead of checking on the computer, one usually has to call down to find the results. Still, each day, Jenny will come in after rounds, look up labs on the computer, discover that they aren't posted, and say, "Oh, my God, this is *so* painful! I can't stand it!" Then she'll pick up the phone and call the laboratory.

After lunch, about 2 p.m., she'll try to find one of the social workers to find out if we can send such-and-such a patient to a nursing home. Some of the social workers are excellent; some

---

* At University of Cincinnati, one of the most important roles that the third-years play is to be retrievers of food on call nights. Since we have no pressing patient responsibilities and are relatively free to come and go, we are generally expected to grab dinner for the team if we're not too busy. Almost every student I know is perfectly happy with this arrangement, having what amounts to a one-hour break in the middle of the long, arduous call day.

are truly awful. *All* of the social workers are stretched too thin. Paging them doesn't necessarily guarantee that they'll call you back, but it's the only easy way to track them down. As Jenny punches in the numbers to page a social worker, she will announce that she is doing so but knows they won't call her back. "This place is *so* painful," she'll say.

She's so reliable about this you can almost set your watch by it.

Monday, March 12   post-call

A great deal of our work as medical students is geared toward learning a specialized vocabulary. Some of the "medicalized" words I've been thinking about in the last couple of days are these:

Anasarca and *asterixis*. Good luck if you can pronounce them. When we were on-call last Wednesday night we received a patient from the University who was picked up by Bob. I didn't know what was going on with him, but later in the evening, when I went to check up on one of my patients, I saw Bob and Chris examining him. From the doorway he looked like a typical VA patient—a little disheveled, half-naked, overweight, and beaten up. His arms were extended and he kept flapping his hands down. He put his arms down, and I heard Chris ask him to put his arms out again. He did so, and repeated the flapping motion. I thought it was odd and decided to ask later. Later on, Bob said to me, "Did you get a look at that guy? Man, does he have anasarca! He's blown up like a balloon!"

"Anasarca" is a term used to denote severe edema, which itself is a term used to denote swelling. I only learned the word a couple of months ago, and couldn't understand why they not only needed *edema* but in addition *anasarca* to describe various stages of swelling.

I found out the following morning why someone came up with anasarca. By this time I had learned the patient's name was Mr. Caffrey, and I learned a little of his story. This was a gentleman in his fifties who had a dying liver, in addition to a not especially happy heart and pair of lungs. His knees had been bothering him, and he had ingested an entire bottle of Advil in a few hours. Word to the wise: Ingesting a bottle of Advil isn't being nice to your body. It's being downright nasty if your liver is in the precarious state Mr. Caffrey's was in. First, his kidneys failed, and he retained a large quantity of fluid, developing several fluid-filled sacs on his body, which he initially "treated" by poking with a pin, until he decided that it might not be such a good idea to do this, at which time he went to the VA emergency room.

When we walked in that morning, we saw a man who was not merely bloated. Dr. Lancing, our attending physician, put his stethoscope to Mr. Caffrey's stomach to listen for bowel sounds, and when he withdrew the instrument there was a perfectly round indentation marking the spot, as if he were made of mud, not skin. If you pushed on the skin in one spot long enough, fluid would just seep directly through the skin. When we had him sitting upright, we needed to get him stockings to stop all the drainage going directly through his feet.

Asterixis refers to an unintentional hand-flapping motion Mr. Caffrey made with his hands when he held his arms out. It's a crude test to measure the degree of central nervous system (i.e. brain) involvement in a patient with hepatic failure.

I'm sure that, during my first two years of medical school, I came across the words *anasarca* and *asterixis*. I could have studied those words until I was blue in the face, but I wouldn't have been able to recall their meaning until I had seen it, which I did. Now I will never forget.

Both the asterixis and the anasarca are the result of a dying liver — the liver can't make enough of a protein called *albumin*, and one of albumin's jobs is to hold water inside the vascular system, the "pipes" of the body, as it were. If the water seeps out of the arteries and veins into the tissues of the body, then it can't get to the kidneys, which would excrete it. Thus you can get kidney failure as an added consequence. When we got Mr. Caffrey as a transfer, that's the shape he was in. His kidneys were hardly producing urine, which meant that toxic metabolites in his body weren't being eliminated. Moreover, since his liver wasn't producing enough albumin to keep the water in the vasculature, his blood pressure was dropping, and he wasn't getting enough blood to his vital organs — among which are the liver and kidneys, making the problem difficult to self-correct.

The bottom line was that he was a very sick guy. After we saw him on rounds on Thursday, Dr. Lancing was reviewing with Bob and Chris their plan of action, which was basically to restrict his fluid intake and give him some diuretics (to help him urinate away some of the excess fluid), although that appeared not to be doing much good. "So that's it?" I asked. "I mean, what are we going to do for him?"

"Watch him die," Lancing said to me slowly and unblinkingly. "Watch him die very slowly. This is not going to be pretty."

That was Thursday. He's alive today, and almost miraculously, he will likely leave the hospital under his own power in the coming days. So, for reasons unknown (possibly helped along by the diuretic), his kidneys and liver managed to correct enough so that he could urinate off enough of the excess fluid to become medically stable. As of today, his kidney function is good, and his liver is returning to some degree of normalcy — as much as a cirrhotic liver can return to normal.

❊❊❊❊❊❊❊❊❊

The next word is hits. A "hit" means a new patient pick-up when one is on call, thus: How many hits did you get last night? Obviously patients aren't exactly charmed if they should happen to overhear one of their residents refer to them as a "hit." Whether it's been the source of lawsuits I do not know, but it seems to have caused such grief for attendings that we've been told repeatedly not to call our patients hits. "Don't worry," they have said at the beginning of every rotation. "You'll hear some resident in the elevator talk about how many 'hits' he got on call. Just don't you do it."

Last night, when we were hanging out in the conference room, Bob asked Jenny, "So, has everyone gotten two hits so far?" Because the delivery was so casual, and the response from everyone else in the room so nonchalant, it didn't immediately occur to me what I had just heard.

Word #4 is guaiac. Not "guaiac" the noun, as in "guaiac-positive stools," meaning that there is blood in someone's stool that isn't visible to the naked eye. Pronounced "gwai-ack," you find out if someone has guaiac-positive stools by lubing your glove-covered finger and placing it in the unfortunate patient's rectum, swabbing their stool on a special test paper, applying a solution to the paper, and then waiting to see if there is a reaction (if there is blood, the sample will turn a bluish color). But guaiac, like many, many nouns in medicine, has become a verb—"to guaiac," meaning to administer a rectal examination to check for occult blood. I have to go guaiac that patient before we can put him on heparin, or I've guaiacked six patients today! Something like that.

Guaiac is hardly the only one. To seize in the outside world typically means to grab onto something, like the phrase carpe diem made famous in Dead Poet's Society—seize the day. In medicine, it means to have a seizure. Did the patient seize? is an oft-heard question on rounds or in conferences. Heparin is a blood thinner, but if you receive heparin, you've become heparinized.

Additional words: Nephrons and neurons are the names of basic units of the kidney and brain, respectively. Thus "nephrology" is the medical subspecialty devoted to kidney disease, while "neurology," of course, deals with brain disorders. If you're one of those docs, you're called a "nephrologist" or "neurologist." That is, unless Dr. Lancing is talking about you, in which case you're a "nephron" or "neuron." Thus: "let's get the neurons on board and see what they think." Or: "yeah, I'll have to ask a nephron about that sometime."

Dr. Lancing seems to be something of a Trekkie as well. If I'm not mistaken, he's got a Star Trek crew-member lapel pin which he has on his White Coat. And at the end of the daily morning update, when we get up to physically round on the patients, he says, "Okay, let's go see some humanoids."

☹☹☹☹☹☹☹☹☹

Slowly I can see things changing in terms of my capabilities: Take one of my current patients, George McBarren. It's the first time in medical school where I feel like a patient is truly primarily my responsibility. Jenny's giving me room to work with him, to follow-up with the various services that we're dealing with at the moment, and to talk to him alone. In a meaningful way, I am his doctor.

Unfortunately, what I just told him earlier today when we were alone together was that his right leg may need to come off. He left leg is already amputated above the knee, and his right one has been causing him chronic pain for years, in part because he isn't getting proper blood supply to the lower part of his leg, and in part because he has had an ulcer on his Achilles tendon about 5 x 2 centimeters for a few years and it isn't healing. He's a retired schoolteacher from Chilicothe whose wife died twenty years ago. Last week the pain became unbearable, so yesterday morning he called his neighbor, who took him to Cincinnati to get admitted and see if anything could be done.

We talked the first time down in the ER, and he mentioned to me that several years earlier, when he had the amputation, he spoke with Dr. Gottfried (one of the vascular surgeons). "Gottfried tried to see what I would think about getting an amputation," he said. "He didn't come right out and say it, but he indicated that it might have to happen. I told him it would happen over my dead body!"

We ran some tests this morning to identify the cause of the pain and see if medical (i.e. non-surgical) therapy was going to help, but it was becoming increasingly clear that the underlying cause of the problem was insufficient blood flow from severely narrowed arteries, and no amount of IV antibiotics were going to help if they couldn't be delivered in sufficient quantity through his blood. I talked to the surgery residents after we rounded and they weren't hopeful that the limb could be revascularized. There's a possibility that we can do a balloon-angioplasty (in the same way that they do angioplasties on heart vessels), but in order to get to the surgery, we would have to do an angiogram, and they are doubtful that that would take place given the risks of the procedure.

That's where we were at with him at approximately noon today, and I thought to myself that if he's going to absolutely resist the idea of an amputation, it may well be over his dead body. I talked about it with Jenny and she told me that I should talk to him and see what he thought about his options. So I did. I've been in medical school for three years, and it was the first time I had ever truly felt like a doctor. I had to go to a patient's room and find out what he thought about the fact that the only thing we may be able to do for him is remove his leg. I wasn't just writing notes for practice or learning how to do the best physical exam, but I was coordinating a patient's care, and if I fucked up he was not going to get the care that he deserved.

The conversation went a good deal better than I had anticipated. Given his remark the day before in the ER, my impression was that he was going to shout, to rail against me, to tell me to go to hell if I try to sell him on an amputation. I explained to him that we were running some tests so that we could develop a game plan, but we had talked with the surgeons and they were concerned that we might not be able to solve the problem in his leg, and they've indicated to us that they may recommend an amputation.

He looked at me with sad but resigned eyes, but there was no hint of hostility. "I thought it would come to this," he said. "I figured that one day I'd end up in the nursing home. You know, because if I get the amputation I'm not going to be able to get around for myself in my home. At least now, with this leg, even in the shape it's in, I can get around, cook for myself, use the commode that I've set up. I drive places with a prosthesis for the other leg. But I thought it would come to this.

"I'm hopeful, though. I'm going to think positive thoughts. You're going to try to save it, aren't you?"

"Oh, yes, of course we are," I said. "This isn't our plan right now. I just wanted to see how you felt about it if it comes to that."

Later I relayed the conversation to Chris. "Oh, he's worried about having to go to a nursing home?" he said. "Well, that's something we can do something about, because I don't think that it's a definite that he has to move out." He was about to add something, then just looked at me and said, "we'll talk about this more tomorrow. In the meantime, you're done today, so get out of here."

Tuesday, March 13

In medicine, doctors, especially the male ones, have long attempted to compensate for the fact that they weren't getting all the chicks, who instead were worshipping jocks, by naming medical things after themselves. You've got the Zollinger-Ellison Syndrome, the ligament of Treitz, the DeBakey clamp, the Levine Sign, and the list goes on and on. This practice is considerably more rare than it was a few generations ago, but you still see it pop up occasionally.

Today, Bob Struggins made his addition to eponymous medical jargon when trying to justify to Jerrold why one of his patients should be discharged. "I know he's ready to go," said Bob, despite the fact that his labs that morning did not indicate any substantial improvement.

"Why's that?" asked Dr. Lancing.

"He's got a positive Struggins Sign."

"What's that?" Chris Szymanowski asked.

"It's the sign that a vet is okay to go home when he can get out of his bed, in his little Johnnie gown, walk all the way down the hall, take the elevator to the first floor, and go outside in thirty-degree weather to smoke cigarettes."

"That sounds reasonable. Start the paperwork for discharge," Dr. Lancing said.

Wednesday, March 14   pre-call

We had "Marning Rounds" today. Dr. Marning is about

70 years old, is one of the senior members of the department, and does small-group educational sessions with the Medicine students (in our case, his small group was just the four of us over at the VA this month). People *adore* him. They speak of him like he's a myth. With all that hype, I was afraid that he wasn't going to be up to the billing. He was quite refreshing, though, and I was glad I got to spend an hour with him looking at blood slides while he peppered his discussion of his favorite restaurants in California. At least he had personality, and I shared his love of good food.

At one point, he was discussing a disease called idiopathic thrombocytopenic purpura, or ITP for short. It's a disease in which your blood platelets — little guys that help form blood clots — get reduced to extremely dangerous levels. While looking at an ITP slide and discussing the patient's history, Marning mentioned the treatment they gave the patient was plasmapheresis, i.e. filtering the blood.

"Um, what are they plasmapheres*ing*?" I asked.

Dr. Marning looked at me and smiled. "You know, the truth is that we don't really know. That's a very good question, very observant of you."

Chastity, one of my classmates, looked at me and smiled and whispered *very good*. "Oh, I'm just revved up from the crack I took this morning," I whispered back.

"What's that?" Marning said.

"Ahem," clearing my throat — "Just had my stimulants, Doctor Marning," I said.

"Oh, that's okay. Nothing like a good cup of coffee to start the day off."

Sunday, March 18   pre-call

Code Blue is a full-out emergency in which every available doc in the hospital carrying a "code pager" must drop whatever he or she is doing and hustle to the site of the emergency. Codes are meant for people who are in imminent danger of dying, but the two times I was called to a code blue at the VA this was not the case. Once a very drunk vet sprawled out across the cafeteria floor and someone panicked; the second time a vet in the ophthalmology clinic got up from his chair too quickly and fainted, and again a not-too-cool-headed person hit the code button.

When a code is called about ten or twenty people come running from all corners of the hospital. For my part, being just a medical student and not being "truly" responsible for patients' lives, this is more of a fun exercise than it is a real nerve-wracking time. When we got to these "codes," however, the docs who *were* sweating it out were none-too-pleased when they discovered the non-emergent nature of the situation. People walked away, grumbling enough to be heard.

Code Brown is the unofficial name applied to the smell of feces that sometimes drifts into the hallways when a patient has become sick or soiled himself. The other morning, we went to start rounds near the Respiratory Care and Cardiac Care Units. A distinctly unpleasant odor hung in the air. "Oh my God, Code Brown!" said Bob. Jenny concurred, while Mina, Katrina and I said nothing. Jenny and Bob prevailed upon Chris to move the proceedings to somewhere more odoristically pleasant.

Code Green is the official name applied to a psych patient who has managed to escape the psych floor and is at risk for flight from the hospital. It's not very hard to escape from the Psych Ward (situated on the 7th floor of the 9-story hospital), as patients are walking in and out all the time to take a smoke, and the staff isn't hyper-vigilant about monitoring which patients are coming and going. Sometimes one of the patients who does not have "smoking privileges" goes AWOL, and that's where the Code Green comes in.

So Friday I'm walking down the hallway of the 5th floor minding my own business. I'm post-call so I'm wearing my scrubs, and I see a nurse slowly walking after someone who's clearly a patient, and an agitated-looking one at that. No one else is near them. A lab tech who happened to be in the hall looks at me and says, "Hey, that guy's a psych patient and he's trying to leave the hospital — go help her!"

Two seconds later my pager sounds the Code Green. So I leap into action. I've dealt with psych patients before, and as psych emergencies go this one seemed pretty tame, since he wasn't violent, wasn't throwing anything, wasn't making any threats or acting in any way that could be construed as intimidating. The nurse was doing her best to keep him calm and re-directed so that he wouldn't leave the hospital but instead would return to the psych ward. I came over mostly to keep an eye on the guy and prevent him from going anywhere before the psych personnel arrived. It was a fairly easy job.

"Hey there, guy," I said. "Listen, what's going on? What's the matter?"

"I'm getting out of here," he said as he pressed the elevator button. The nurse stepped in front of the elevator door just in case it opened, which, given the efficiency of the VA elevators, wasn't likely to happen momentarily. "I've got to go downtown and pick up my furniture from my house," he added.

"You don't *have* a house," the nurse gently reminded him.

"Now how do you know that?" he snapped back.

"Well, why don't we head back to the ward so we can straighten this out, okay?" I said. "If your furniture's there, it won't mind if you took an extra half hour to work everything out with us."

He studied me, and turned away from the elevator to address me. "You've got to understand, I *want* my furniture. I've got to go pick it up."

"That sounds perfectly reasonable. Let's just make sure that you're safe to leave, because I'm not sure you should be going right at this moment." I had managed to get within two feet of him, and extended my hand around his shoulder. He didn't resist, and I thought that, as the nurse took him by the other arm, we had easily and painlessly resolved this problem.

At that moment, one of the VA security police wheeled around the corner. He was a short, fat man, wearing thick square steel-rimmed glasses, with a cherry-red nose produced from years of drinking. From appearances, soon he could be one of the VA patients *himself*. He looked at the man, squared his shoulders, and grabbed his walkie-talkie.

"Yeah, this is Officer Roush, on the scene at the Code Green. We're on the seventh floor Elevator Bay B, and we will have the AWOL returned shortly. Over." He then took two steps toward the patient. "Step *away* from the elevator door and drop that bag right *now!*" he snapped.

The nurse and I quickly exchanged glances. "Um, we've got things under control here," I said, but in the two seconds that I managed to say this, the patient had caught and processed the full dose of the cop's hatred, and all hell broke loose.

"I'm gonna *fucking* go to my home and get my furniture! I need to get on the bus *now!*" He held tightly to his "bag," a little fanny-pack that probably held such extremely dangerous items as a toothbrush and comb, and the cop took a step closer.

"Could you let us handle this?" the nurse asked. By this point the man had begun to scream like a banshee while retreating from the cop, who was advancing toward him. There wasn't much room in the corridor, and at that moment I thought that what had started out as an almost charming AWOL moment was going to become violent, and my experiences in psychiatry had underscored to me that when a psych patient—even a thin, weak patient—feels threatened, he can become very dangerous indeed.

Several large orderlies had come around the corner, so that what started out as three people accidentally thrust together by circumstances who decided to take a walk together was about to turn into a melee. I realized that my presence made no difference at that point, and decided to return to my work of checking labs and writing notes. As I parted through the group I caught eyes with one of the orderlies, a large black guy who was likely going to be called upon shortly to pounce on the unfortunate man, still screaming away at Officer Roush, who kept fueling the fire.

"What the fuck is the matter with that cop?" I asked the orderly, with the intent of being loud enough so that everyone could hear me. "I mean, we had this guy perfectly calm and then he comes along with his John Wayne act and now we've got *this!*"

The orderly laughed. "Oh, that's John Roush," he explained. "He's stuck being a security guard at the VA, you know? But he wants to be a big, tough guy, so he pounces on something like this. I've ended up being called into these situations more times that I can remember. This happens a few times a month."

"Well, he's a mother fucking liability," I said. "Someone needs to can that man's ass."

Thursday, March 22

Today was Match Day.

Match Day is arguably the most important day of a medical student's life. It's only slightly less important than the day you actually get *accepted* to medical school. The Match represents the end of a very grueling process similar to the med school application process. The main difference is that if the med school application process doesn't go well, you don't get to be a doctor at all; even if the Match doesn't go well, you'll almost certainly still be some kind of doctor, and unless you are seeking a job in one of the most competitive fields, you'll likely get to be the kind of doctor you want to be. Your chances of getting into medical school at the turn of the 21st century are roughly one in three. Yet as a student at a US medical school, your chances of matching for residency are better than *98 percent*. In essence, there are only two ways you cannot match as a US medical grad. One is to be an absolutely, widely-recognized horrible medical student that no program, even one desperate for help, wants to take you on as a liability. The other, more common way is to be one who shoots too high in too competitive a specialty, without a backup plan.

There's another difference between getting into medical school and matching: You can get many medical school acceptances, but you get only *one* match. For instance, say you've applied to 20 places for admission to med school. Five reject you outright, and you send so-called "secondary applications" to the remaining fifteen. Ten select you for an interview. You interview at all of them, and over the coming months five acceptances trickle back. You sit down and compare all of the schools to which you have been accepted, taking cost, prestige, location, and anything else into consideration. In the end, it's *your* choice which of those five schools you attend, and you can keep the schools hanging on the line until mid-May, when you finally have to commit to just one. All things considered, it's a very advantageous system for those who manage to make the cut, because students accepted to several med schools dictate where they will attend.

But now you're doing the Match for residency. Like before, you send out 20 applications and get 10 interviews. After the interviews, you rank, from first to last, the programs that you want to get into for your residency. At the same time, each program sits down at the end of interview season and places *you* in a rank list. Everyone's lists (hospitals and students) are due in mid-February, and all the lists are placed together into a massive computer program, which proceeds to "match" the residency program's top choices to the applicants' top choices. After the program runs, every medical student who matches has *one* program name. Barring unusual circumstances, they are obligated to attend this program for residency.

Here are some rough match numbers to give you an idea of what's at stake: There are nearly 17,000 US medical students participating in the match, while there are about 22,000 residency positions available. *This* is why it's very difficult not to match. What do programs do for those other 5,000 positions? They seek the roughly 25,000 Foreign Medical Grads (officially called "International Medical Graduates," or IMGs) who are also participating in the match. These 25,000 include Canadian medical grads, European medical grads, US citizens who attended Carribean or Mexican medical schools, the occasional Chinese medical doc, and what appears to me to be one of the most significant groups, the Indian and Pakistani medical grads and docs.

If you *don't* match, the schools will be notified 72 hours prior to the official announcement of the Match, which is Thursday at noon, Eastern Time. The schools will then get in touch with you to let you know you didn't match, at which point you enter into a nasty frenzy called "the scramble." In the scramble, all of the programs that did not fully match (i.e. there were open residency slots because not enough applicants had ranked them) are seeking people, and students who haven't matched are seeking a program.

I had originally thought that the scramble was a process that lasted a few weeks, during which time you interviewed at programs, judiciously weighing the merits of one program over the other. I was rudely disabused of this notion earlier today, when I ran into a few of the fourth-years that I knew. I was chatting with them, asking them where they matched, and the topic turned to the scramble. I must have said something about the scramblees not yet knowing what they were going to do next year, because I saw several confused glances being returned to me. "Steven, the scramble is over already," said one of the students.

So it was. In those 72 hours between the announcement of the non-matched students and the formal announcement of the Match results, the scramble takes place almost entirely by phone, and it must occur at a feverish pace. Every program is trying to pick up every available slot to fill its manpower requirement, and every student who doesn't match is trying to get a job somewhere, *any*where, and preferably in their desired specialty. Sometimes the luck may run your way, and you might find a plum spot at a great hospital that went unfilled for whatever reason. But you better talk to the program director mighty quick, because there's dozens of other medical school deans across the country that are chomping at the bit to talk to the same program director in order to extol the virtues of their three unmatched candidates.

What I know of the Match numbers this year more or less has come from a long, alcohol-soaked evening with Vikash and Bob "Scrub" Beatty. Bob and Vikash informed me that, nationwide, nearly 25 percent of those students trying to match in radiology were rejected, that only 10 percent of those going after neurosurgery came up empty-handed, and that there were dozens of programs in general surgery that had openings (apparently this was something previously unheard of). Anesthesia, a specialty that only a year or two ago was dying to grab qualified residents, filled many of its residency slots, speculation being that it may be on the upswing in terms of desirability.

As far as UC goes, there were about a half-dozen students who had to scramble. One of them was a guy named Brian who was working on the endocrine consult team down at the VA, and I was working with him on my patient, Mr. Jorgens, a 26 year-old with Type I diabetes. On Monday, Brian got paged by the Dean as we were discussing the patient's case. One of his classmates looked at him, and he quietly got up and said, "gotta go up the hill to talk to the Dean," and the room got so quiet you could hear the proverbial pin drop. Brian was going to scramble.

At any rate, on Tuesday, I needed to touch base with him about my patient, and the Endocrine Fellow wasn't returning my pages. So I tried to page the VA operator to find out Brian's pager number, and that got me nowhere. The only person I knew who would know his pager number was the Dean, so I gave her a call, totally unaware of the role she was playing in helping students scramble, and equally unaware that students scrambled the day after they failed to match.

"Hi," I started out on the phone—how I managed to get through to her office on such a day is an open question—"listen, there's a fourth-year who's working on the Endocrine Team down here at the VA, and I was wondering if you might have his pager number since I can't manage to track him down."

"Well, what's his name?" she asked me.

"Oh, it's Brian MacDougal," I said.

"It's funny you should say that, Steven, because he's standing right here."

"*He is?*"

"Yes he is, and I can *assure* you that what he's doing here is more important right now than what you need to ask him, but let me see if he'll talk to you."

Woops. I had no idea that the scramble occurred with that kind of urgency.

It is one of the central ironies of American medicine at the end of the 20th century that many of the most accomplished medical students pursue the least demanding residencies.

Brian is going to graduate in the top quarter of his class, as are *most* of those who failed to match. This is because they were trying to match into Radiology, the hot-hot-hot field of the past few years.

Now, broadly speaking, radiology isn't very challenging in terms of patient care. There are a few radiologists involved in something known as "interventional radiology" who perform invasive procedures on patients — think of it as "surgery lite" and you've got a rough idea of it. Interventional radiology is a more demanding field, not least because people can die beneath your fingers due to the riskiness of the procedures. But as I said, there aren't a lot of those folks walking around. Most practicing radiologists spend their time sitting in caves staring at films and dictating what they see. All in all, it's not one of the most scintillating fields in terms of requiring a wide breadth of medical knowledge, and it further requires little social skills since there's little interaction with patients.

Orthopedic Surgery, another one of the super-competitive residency programs, isn't very challenging either. "When I was in medical school, we used to think that Ortho was a field for dumb jocks," one doctor who had graduated in the 70s confided to me. "Now it's considered such a desirable field, and lots of good people are going into it. But seriously, how complicated can *bones* be?"

Neither is Dermatology, which is almost perennially the single most competitive residency as measured by percentage of people who fail to match (usually one-quarter to one-third of people don't make the cut). Derm is highly competitive for many reasons: It involves virtually no call — even as a resident. The patients are usually very healthy, and are deeply grateful when you help clear their zits up. No patient is going to thank a medicine doc for giving them a drug that will prevent a heart attack they can't feel — but the patient certainly *will* appreciate the abdominal discomfort and diarrhea the drug produces. By contrast, a derm patient comes in with a mildly disfigured face that causes severe embarrassment, and after a topical drug — *poof!* No more facial nasties. Your patients will *love* you. What kind of med student wouldn't want that?

But seriously, how complicated can *skin* be? How much are you sweating to keep patients from the brink of death? You aren't at all, except in the rare circumstance when you're dealing with a late-stage melanoma patient, in which case you've probably punted the problem to an oncologist or a surgeon anyway, or if you stumble across a case of Stevens-Johnson syndrome, a nasty condition in which the skin basically says, "I quit," and the patients end up in the burn unit, fighting for their lives. In that case, the Intensive Care people are dealing with the situation, and as a dermatologist you pretty much let them handle the crisis.

At the other end of the spectrum, the hardest working people in the biz, the general surgeons, are suffering from a period of waning interest. Applications to general surgery, which 20 to 30 years ago was among the most competitive fields, have been going down for nearly a decade, and the non-match rate, which used to be over 20 percent, is now about five. It's still a relatively competitive field, but it's much easier to become a surgeon today than ever before. General surgeons are a bit like the über-people of surgery: Obstetrics and gynecology, also a surgical field, is not quite as competitive as general surgery, but still competitive on a relative scale.

Fields that aren't competitive include the biggies: Medicine, pediatrics, and family medicine. Those three fields account for just under half of the positions of all those who match, and consequently you're pretty much a shoo-in if you want to be a kiddie doc. Whether or not you'll make the cut at CHOP — the Children's Hospital of Philadelphia, one of the most renowned, and thus competitive, programs in pediatrics — is less certain, but there are plenty of good programs out there looking for decent candidates. As a US medical grad you'll almost certainly match in medicine; the only question is whether you'll get into a slightly more competitive "academic" program based at a major University medical center, or if you'll settle for a less competitive "private" program where your teachers are practicing docs, not part-time docs who do lots of research.

These fields are less competitive largely because of one reason: Money. General surgeons work very, very hard, but they also earn about twice that of a family doc. Even within medicine, the more lucrative the field, the more competitive: The two subspecialties with the highest incomes, GI and cardiology, also are the only two where you might not be able to match into fellowship. Virtually all other subspecialties in internal medicine are hurting for qualified, interested people, and this is due to the fact that you don't earn more as an ID doc than you do as a general internist. Why on earth would you bother to spend three extra years at one-third the salary of your peers, only to enter into a job that doesn't earn more bucks?

The three of us were reviewing all this, sitting in Mecklenberg drinking our beer, wondering about what the future holds. Bob is bound for neurosurgery, and he was heartened by this year's numbers; he feels like he has a legitimate shot at getting into a decent neurosurgery program next year, which is good, given that neurosurgery is not a specialty that has an easy backup. Meaning that if you don't match into highly-competitive plastic surgery, there's always general surgery; or if you don't match into general surgery, there's always ER or OB/GYN, which involves a lot of surgery and procedures. If you can't match into medicine (though this is almost impossible), there's always Family Medicine, about the least competitive field out there. But if your heart is set on neurosurgery, neither neurology nor general surgery are really good backups, because neuro involves few procedures if any, while brain and spine surgery is totally different from all other kinds of surgeries (while the difference between general and gynecologic surgery is far less profound). So Bob had reason for cheer.

Vikash hasn't made his mind up. He might want to be a urologist, or he might want to be a general surgeon. Then again, he might want to go into medicine with an eye toward GI or Cards. He likes procedures, but he doesn't really want to spend his professional life working like a slave, so for that reason he's less enamored of general surgery and cardiology. But getting into urology—a 9-to5 surgical specialty—is a crapshoot (only 200 positions available in the US each year), and GI has recently become perhaps the most competitive subspecialty in medicine. So he's not sure where he stands at the moment, trying to balance his desire to be in a surgical field with his desire for a good quality of life.

As for me, I'm on the fence between peds and medicine. Because neither field is especially competitive, I'm not too concerned about not matching, and my guess is that I'll match into a decent program. The question I keep asking myself is which kind of doc do I *want* to be? In internal medicine, you deal with a lot of chronic problems to which there are, at present, no really good solutions. Oh, sure, you can stent a blocked coronary artery or you can control someone's diabetes or hypertension with various medications, but often these are only stalling measures. Moreover, given the unwillingness of many patients to comply with medication regimens that have unpleasant side effects, you often fight a losing battle.

Peds is a different beast entirely. One doc described it this way: "Listen, you'll see a lot of patients in internal medicine who'll be crying about their slightly arthritic elbow — 'ooh, doc, it hurts so much!' — like it's the end of the world. Me, I'll come and see a kid who's got something really terrible going on with him, like cancer or a broken bone, and he's trying to get out of this exam as soon as possible so that he can go outside and play baseball! I'd rather deal with the kid, you know?"

I know, I know. But how much of the touchy-feely side of pediatrics will I be able to handle before I toss my cookies? There's a meeting scheduled on April 4 at Children's for those who are thinking about pediatrics, hosted by the director of the residency program, and I'll see how things pan out once I attend. Maybe there will be some new insights that I will have once I hear the pitch.

Wednesday, March 28 post-call

Just came back from shooting baskets with some 12 year-old to help get my mind off of the hospital. I saw my first *genuine* code last night — in fact, was intimately involved in it — and although I'm perfectly calm about it now, it was a relatively emotionally jarring situation when it happened. I know that I've referred in the past to the feeling I've gotten when a code is called—a bit of *whee!* because you get to run through the hospital and feel like you're an actor in ER.

The line "when a code is called, the first thing to do is check your own pulse" doesn't hold true for a third-year student, who has no responsibilities. Yet the moment I entered Mr. Caffrey's door I knew that I wasn't going to feel good ever again about codes, because I learned what the "real" docs and nurses have long known: That a code is often another way of saying "this patient is about to die, come quick."

You remember Mr. Caffrey, the gentleman with the liver and kidneys teetering on the brink of oblivion. Although Dr. Lancing had predicted that we would watch him die a slow death, he managed to bounce back. His kidneys miraculously recovered, and using a drug called lasix, we were able to get his kidneys to clear off an enormous volume of fluid that had been building up and was poised to drown him from the inside out. We sent him home and considered ourselves lucky. About a week later, though, he returned to our service. Once admitted, the plan for him was the same as before: Drain fluid and hope for the best.

We got the code at 2:30 a.m. I had gone to sleep only fifteen minutes earlier, because I had to stay up to check on the cardiac enzymes for one of my patients. The pager went off, and announced the room. It didn't ring any bells, and as I walked out into the hallway, I saw Katrina come out. We took off down the back stairs from the 9th floor, only to realize as we got to the 6th that that floor was locked, so we went to the 5th, came out, doubled back to the main staircase, ran up, and bolted for the room.

When I came into the room, it seemed like bedlam. Mr. Caffrey was lying there, looking terribly bloated and completely naked, with a catheter sticking out of his penis and various IV lines in his arms. There were approximately fifteen people there, about six of whom were physically attending to Mr. Caffrey, with the remainder just standing at the periphery of the room looking on. I was originally part of this group, not about to do anything until I had a direct order to do so, which didn't take long. Kelley, an intern who was working in the Intensive Care Unit, was trying to give the very large Mr. Caffrey chest compressions, but she was too short and didn't have the upper-body strength. I was the tallest person in the room, and her eyes (and those of a few others) fell upon me. So I stepped up to the plate, moved into her position, put my two hands smack on his sternum the way I had trained to do *two years* earlier, and started doing compressions. My adrenaline at that point was running too high to be nervous or self-conscious about doing it.

"Dude, don't just start going at it," said Chris. Chris, being the senior medicine resident in the hospital at that moment, was running the code. He grabbed my hand, said, "make sure you find the xiphoid and move *up* from it. You don't want to be pushing in his xiphoid. Get on the sternum." I repositioned my hand, remembering the technique I had been taught so long ago, and started compressing.

After four minutes of this, Chris looks at me and says, "Hey, this guy needs to get gloved. Let someone else take over right now." In the heat of the moment, I forgot to put my latex gloves on. It wasn't a critical error in this situation (there are other cases in which it would be a tremendous error to forget to glove; in this case, Mr. Caffrey wasn't bleeding and wasn't known to have HIV, or Hepatitis B or C), so I stepped back and let Bob take over while I put some gloves on. Meanwhile the room was a whirlwind of activity; Chris would call out for lidocaine, or epinephrine, there would be some scrambling, opening of drawers on the "crash cart" used for coding patients, and then the drug would be produced and injected into Mr. Caffrey.

By the time I returned to the bedside only a few minutes later (by this time it was about 2:55), it was becoming clear to me that he wasn't going to make it. He had been in a state known as PEA, or "pulseless electric activity," and Chris was asking how long the code had been running. As I pushed on his chest, I stared down into his wide open eyes, his mouth holding the tube used to force air into his lungs. He looked kind of surprised by the whole thing. Yet he wasn't surprised at all; he was dead.

"Guys, what's it been?" Chris asked.

"Thirty minutes," one of the nurses said.

"That's it. Let's call it."

And that was it. The room instantly emptied of extra personnel, and those of us who had been working on Mr. Caffrey, now covered with our own sweat or his body fluids, made our way over to the sink to wash ourselves, and the nursing team swung into action to make Mr. Caffrey presentable. We walked out into the hallway, and Chris and Bob were talking about filling out the death note and calling his son. I just stood there, shaking like a leaf, feeling partly like I needed to vomit and partly like I needed to cry. Doing my best to suppress both, I headed back to my call room and laid in bed, wide awake for the next two hours.

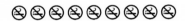

Mr. Parsons is a patient of mine with new-onset congestive heart failure. Until now, he had been a very healthy gentleman in his mid-70s who exercised daily, tended his garden, and puttered around his house, though he still ate the standard vet diet consisting almost exclusively of eggs, potatoes, and meat. He had come in feeling tired and short of breath. On physical exam even *I* could tell he had a great deal of fluid in his lungs — the sound when you place a stethoscope on his back is a bit like listening to crinkling paper, the sound of air trying to rush into lungs that the fluid has collapsed. How this had happened so suddenly was a matter of concern, since he could likely have infarcted a large section of his heart (that is, had a massive but "silent" heart attack).

During rounds in the morning, as we were going over his history, physical, and laboratories (negative for a heart attack), Dr. Lancing said that Parsons should go to the cardiac catheterization lab. A cath is a routine procedure, and generally pretty safe, but it's not without its risks. As it turned out, his roommate, also a patient under our care, had gone to the cath lab the day before and developed something called ventricular fibrillation, and he had to be shocked to be revived. Ultimately, the man did fine.

By the time we had come to the room to explain to Mr. Parsons that he needed a cath, though, he had had a long discussion with his roomie about *his* experiences in the lab. We were unaware of this when Lancing said, "Mr. Parsons, we've been looking at your labs and we really think a catheterization is the best test for you. How do you feel about that?"

Mr. Parsons had smiled a very nice, warm smile, like he hadn't wanted to offend us, but he shook his head. "You know, doc, I just don't think it's the right test for me. I, uh, don't really want to go to a test and not come back."

This was a very unusual attitude for a vet, since vets typically just shrug when asked about performing tests. *You guys are the docs,* is something like the attitude, *you know what's best, so do it.* For this reason, vets are often popular for residents eager to get experience performing procedures, particularly the surgery crew, who often get to lead the less complicated surgeries.

Lancing nodded. "I take it you heard about Mr. Billingham's experience yesterday."

"Oh yes. Doc, that's not for me."

"Okay. You do understand, though, that's a very rare complication."

He just kept shaking his head, smiling all the while, as if he was hoping this conversation would end very soon.

"Do you understand that an angiogram is probably the best test for you right now?"

"Doc, I just don't want to do it."

"Okay," Lancing said. "Is it possible for us to perform another test? One where we don't have to put big, long catheters in you? We're just going to put you on a treadmill, have you drink some special fluids to help us look at your heart, and take some pictures of it. There's nothing invasive about it at all. What do you think?"

"I suppose that's okay," he said, and we left to make arrangements for him to get a nuclear stress test.

"It's not going to be the greatest test, since we're not going to get a really good look at his coronary anatomy," Lancing said outside. "But it's better than nothing. I'm just worried about what's going to happen if the test shows that there's some reversible ischemia in a portion of his heart, because then the only way we can treat him is to get him into the cath lab."

Later that afternoon, we got the results, and that turned out not to be the case. Mr. Parsons had an almost entirely dead left ventricle. The cardiac cath wouldn't be needed; there wasn't anything further we could do for him, because you can't stent an artery to tissue that's already dead. From here on out, the trick for Mr. Parsons was going to be to keep his fluid intake low enough so that he doesn't flood his lungs, because his dying heart can't pump enough blood to his body, and it backs up into his lungs, causing him to slowly drown. However, we can't give him too little fluid, because he'll dehydrate and possibly kill his kidneys. It's going to be a delicate balancing act, and the life of this gentleman, who had been so vigorous up until now, is going to change dramatically.

Friday, March 30

My conversation yesterday with one of the doctors who directs the medical student education in internal medicine:

"Um, Doctor Smith?"

"Yes, Steven."

"Um, I wanted to check on the policy of taking call on the transition weekend between the inpatient and outpatient months. Uh, you see, I'm finishing my inpatient rotation, and my team takes call on Saturday. I have been told that we're off officially as of Friday at noon, but I also heard that we're not off until Sunday. So, uh, I just wanted to see what the story was."

"The policy is that if you don't have weekend call, you are off Friday at noon. If you have weekend call, you take it."

"Oh." With an emotional thud that I couldn't conceal.

"Think of it this way. You get yet another chance to learn all about medicine."

Hmmm. Think of it this way: My wife doesn't remember my name anymore.

My conversation later that day with Chris:

"Dude, we need to sit down with you and get your evaluation done before you take off."

"Can it wait until Saturday, Chris? It should be slow in the morning."

"What do you mean, 'Saturday'?"

"I'm supposed to take call. I asked Dr. Smith."

"Now why the hell did you do that? Listen, just keep your mouth shut and don't broadcast anything up there to those people. You'll come in Saturday morning, round on your patients, and if we don't get hit by one or two you can get us some lunch and get out of Dodge. We'll do your evaluation then, you idiot."

"Yeah, uh, that sounds good to me."

"I can't believe you told Smith."

Wednesday, April 4

Finally, I can state with near-certainty what kind of a doctor I am going to be. Barring the highly unlikely circumstance that I fall head-over-heels in love with obstetrics and gynecology, my future field is medicine.

The informational meeting for medical students interested in pediatrics was today. Meetings in medical centers almost always start late, but I am an obsessively punctual person, and I arrived at ten-to-four and sat in the pediatric resident conference room waiting for my classmates and the residency director to arrive. Over the coming minutes, several classmates arrived and we began chit-chatting about liking peds, how impressed we were with the Children's Hospital and the peds faculty, and where we might want to go for residency.

Yet as I engaged in these brief conversations, something felt very hollow, like I was *pretending* to be interested in doing a peds residency, but it was just a put-on. I couldn't put my finger on it then and, with the perspective of two whole hours, I can't put my finger on it now. But by the time the director arrived at five past, I had decided to leave. There wasn't any point in listening to the pitch. It felt wrong, and for the first time this year I felt like I *knew* what I would be doing after I graduated. I was going into medicine.

Thursday, April 5

I finished the inpatient rotation on Saturday at about two, after having retrieved lunch one last time for the team. We never picked up a new patient in the morning, so I just finished working on my "off-service" note for a patient.* Dr. Lancing took each of us back to his office in the cardiology suite to present us with our evaluations. Mine was, as usual, on the border between high pass and honors. I got the impression from Lancing that while both he and Chris gave me high marks, there may have been a dispute as to whether I deserved "fours" or "fives." No matter; they're both flattering assessments.

As I finished talking to Lancing about my evaluation, I asked him if he would feel comfortable writing me a letter of recommendation for residency. "Do you need one already?" he said to me.

"Oh, no, I don't, but I'll probably need one in August, which is right around the corner, and I figured I'd just ask now to gauge how you felt about it."

"Yeah, that's no problem. Man, not only will I write you a letter of recommendation, I'll write one that will actually *help* you get into a residency."

Thank *you*, dude.

By the end of the month, I probably most enjoyed hanging out with Bob Struggins, the budding radiologist. Although I was initially put off by his hyper-conservative exterior, I

---

* An off-service note is written in lieu of a discharge summary, when the patient remains in the hospital after the medical team leaves and all the residents and attendings move on to different rotations. Thus it's a summary designed to convey all the pertinent information about the patient's hospital course to the residents who will be taking over his care. In my patient's case, there was a *lot* of information to convey since his was a relatively complicated situation, so it took the better part of the morning to write it, and I had begun it from home the night before.

realized how laid-back and friendly he was, and halfway through the month he was regularly giving me valuable advice about how best to succeed during the AI months, and how to do little things that will help your chances out in the residency dance. We would kid around about the VA patients and their penchant for smoking, even as they were knocking on death's door. We laughed only because there was nothing else to do, given the somewhat depressing scene of watching guys with stumps of legs and various ports sticking into veins in the neck and arms wheeling and hobbling their way toward the outside, the great smoking Mecca, where they could attain a few moments of peace with a few puffs.

I had also come to enjoy working with Mina, and towards the end I became convinced that, although she was clearly behind the curve in terms of her medical education on a few key points, she was going to do well as a doc. We spoke at one point about her career goals when taking call last Tuesday, and she indicated that maybe she wanted to do medicine instead of psych. I told her if that was the case, she should talk to Gene Rouleaux, the Medicine residency director at UC, and that maybe there was a spot open in the second-year roster. It seemed to me that if she had the desire, she should try and hustle to get a spot if there was one to be got.

Leaving the inpatient ward team is a little like leaving a family — even if you are just the "family pet." You may not like your family all the time, but you are with them so often and in such close confines that an inpatient month can't help but be an emotionally intense experience. The outpatient portion of the course, as I learned from pediatrics, is easier — there are fewer expectations on you, so you have more time to relax, to study, to absorb what's happening to you. This definitely has its place, but I prefer the energy and bustle of the hospital.

"After all I've seen, I can tell you this: When it's time for me to have a baby, I'm going straight to the OR to have a C-section."
— Ellie Stern, MD, OB intern

<u>seven</u>

the epidural quarterbacks of OB/GYN

Sunday, April 29

I didn't write much during my outpatient month of internal medicine. It was pretty much a lazy month in terms of working and writing — at least until the last two weeks, when I poured it on as much as I could to study for the exam. How the exam went is an open question. During the morning exam, I became a little giddy after about question 35 or 40, because I was feeling pretty confident that I knew the answer to *every* question that had been thrown at me. *My god!* I started thinking to myself. *I might actually ace this exam!* Then the bottom fell out, and the next sixty-or-so questions were a downhill ride.

But I got a bit ahead of myself there, jumping from April 5 all the way to the test on the 27th without hitting at least some of the highlights in-between. The medicine outpatient rotation involved three half-days with my outpatient-preceptor, Dr. Raymond Dart, who played the same role as Dr. Mittleschmertz in Family Medicine and Dr. Blumstein in Pediatrics. I spent three half-days at the VA student clinic (in which the patients invariably failed to show up), and another half-day working with the nephrologists (kidney docs) down at the VA as part of a sub-specialty rotation.

I dug the nephrologists, who were all incredibly smart and unimposing. One day we were swamped with patients, trying to keep up with the pace so that everyone could be seen without great delay. One of the patients who came to the clinic was in an especially foul mood, and griped from the moment I walked in the door, telling me how pissed he was that he had to wait an hour and a half for his check-up. When I walked back to the doctors' office to present his case, I warned the attending of his disposition. "I don't think you're going to like this," I said after I ran down his medical story. "He's really hot about how long he's waited."

The doctor held the schedule in his hands and perused it. "Well, we were supposed to see him at ten. It's now almost noon. I think he has every right to be upset, and that will be the first thing I tell him," he said. It was the first time I had ever seen a doctor fully acknowledge that it's impolite to keep a patient waiting well beyond their appointment times, and I immediately liked him for his observation, thinking that if one day I don't pursue infectious disease, maybe I could hang out with the kidney guys. They're a pretty cool bunch.

♀♀♀♀♀♀♀♀♀

The really big story of April, however, was my further education in how to do the residency dance, which is now front-and-center in the minds of all third-year students. I spoke with several different people in-the-know about medicine residencies and how to strategize my search. With each new meeting, I became more and more concerned that I would make some misstep at one point or another in the process, and would end up doing a medicine residency in East Podunk Community Hospital.

Applying to residency is a different process than applying to medical school, although not entirely different. Basic rules apply: The more competitive the residency, the more grades & board scores count; likewise, the more competitive the *program* within a residency (Medicine at Brigham & Women's Hospital in Boston vs. Medicine at Christ Hospital in Cincinnati) the more grades & board scores count. But some residency programs place a much higher emphasis than others on those supposed "objective" measures of a student's status: For instance, in many radiology programs, you won't even get your foot in the door if you are not a member of "AOA," or Alpha Omega Alpha, the medical student honors society. On the other hand, some smaller programs in highly competitive residencies like Urology, had only admitted the top smarties into their programs a few years ago, only to discover that they were arrogant or had no social skills, so they actually *avoid* the top students.

(How many Urology programs actually do this is a very open question, but one day during lunch a classmate provided this yarn, so I report it here without any concrete idea of its truth value. But it illustrates another aspect of the residency game, namely, that at least half of the information students obtain about residencies come from other students, regardless of whether the information is true or can even be verified in some meaningful way.)

The real question that every student asks, and what was front-and-center in my mind during the month of April as I began talking to those docs who deal with the residency search, is this: *What are my chances of getting to where I want to go?* I wanted to be in a Medicine program at a major academic medical center in the northeast, preferably in Boston. That meant that there were five programs at the top of my wish list: Mass General, Brigham and Women's, and Beth Israel-Deaconness (all Harvard affiliated); New England Medical Center (Tufts affiliated); and Boston Medical Center (Boston University affiliated).

I first started by posing this question to Gene Rouleaux. The residency director here at UC, Dr. Rouleaux was a logical choice because he was the local expert on what residency programs sought in applicants. He's a gentle man, very soft-spoken, polite, engaging. His lecture to us on the use of evidence-based medicine in the diagnosis of pulmonary embolism was almost completely inscrutable, but this is no matter, especially since I need his help.

After sitting down and exchanging pleasantries, we got down to business, where he asked me some boiler-plate questions about my academic record. "How did you do during the first two years?" he asked.

"A couple of high passes, nothing in honors, no academic trouble."

"And your Step One?"

"Two-nineteen."

"Really? That's good."

"Eh. It's nothing to write home about, but I'm not ashamed of it, I guess."

"And this year?"

Now I puff my chest up. "Honors in Surgery, Psych, and Neuro, high passes in Peds and Oncology, and a pass in that killer course, Family Medicine," I smile wanly. "What can I say?"

He then asked me where I wanted to go, and I named for him the Boston programs, the three big Ohio programs (Case, OSU, and UC), and a couple of New England stragglers like Brown and Dartmouth. After I rattled these programs off, he drew a bell-shaped curve and started writing program names at various points along the curve. At one end of the curve were programs like Yale, Brigham and Women's, Mass General, and Case; at the other end was Brown, Ohio State, and Tufts; and in the middle was UC and Beth Israel-Deaconess.

It struck me as a curious interpretation if it meant what I thought it meant, which was that I should view Brown, OSU, and *Tufts* of all places as safety schools, but as he explained it, I knew I had read the graph correctly. "Why are those three schools safeties?" I asked.

"Because they're not exceptional programs. Ohio State only matched something like five residents last year for their entire department. I've heard that Brown isn't a very strong program. And Tufts is in *serious* financial trouble."

"Really? I thought they had stabilized their situation in the past few years."

"Not from what *I've* heard."

At the other end of the curve were programs that he thought would be tough for me but that I still had a chance at. "And I know the program directors at these places," he said. "When December comes, if you want to get into the Brigham, you let me know and I'll place a call to lobby for you. Residency directors want to know that the people that they're going to get want to go to their program, and I'd be happy to call someone up and say, 'Hey, Steven here *really* wants to be with you.' So let's cross that bridge in December or January."

I felt pretty pumped after leaving that session. Brown, OSU, and Tufts as *safety* schools? Cool! Beth-Israel within my competitive range? Awesome! Here I come, Boston!

About a week later I thought I'd follow up with Mark Silverman, the director of the General Internal Medicine division — the primary-care track of the Medicine department. Silverman, I had learned, spent about a decade at Tufts, so he'd know the lay of the land there. I also figured, since I thought I had made a pretty favorable impression from our case-presentation sessions with him during March, that he might be willing to go to bat for me and make a phone call to a receptive ear.

But the meeting was a polar opposite of the one with Rouleaux. As I recited my academic list to him, he sat in his chair, relaxed, nodding. At the end he looked at me and said politely, "Listen. I don't want to shock you, but I don't think that you'll be competitive at any of the Boston programs with that kind of a record. I think even the weakest programs in Boston expect their applicants to at least have a smattering of honors. I'm not sure what else to say. You might benefit from doing an elective rotation at a program in Boston, but I don't think it's going to make much of a difference."

At that moment, I was certain that my guts were going to come spilling right out. I was so stunned I don't know how I managed to thank him for his candor and excuse myself as gracefully as possible, but I did. Or at least I think I did. I reeled out into the hallway wondering *which* version of my potential corresponded most closely to reality. A *smattering* of honors? Jesus, I had gotten honors in two out of my big three grades thus far! I might well be able to pull off one in Medicine, which leaves OB as a wild card. Theoretically I could get four honors out of the big five, with one high pass. How much better could I do?

An hour or two later I bumped into one of the medicine residents on the elevator, a woman whom I had gotten to know while at the VA in March. I relayed the conversation to her. She wrinkled her nose. "You know, Silverman's such a narrow person," she said. "He's very limited. All he can do is look at the numbers. He's not capable of seeing beyond that. Don't let what he said get to you."

"But what I don't get is how different it was from Gene Rouleaux's assessment," I responded.

"*Well*," she said, "Gene sometimes tends to paint a rosy picture of what's going on. Sometimes *too* rosy. Listen, I think you need to talk to Lana Wasserman. I know that you think she's cold and distant, but try to believe me when I tell you that underneath that formal exterior is someone who really cares about students."

Four days later, I was sitting in Dr. Wasserman's office. Wasserman, the new academic dean, is a cardiologist who did her residency training at Mass General. She has a reputation for having a *very* chilly personality. Would she be of any help? I had gulped, followed the resident's advice, and was now repeating my life's story for the third time in less than two weeks.

Although she didn't say it outright, I inferred that she tended to agree with Silverman. "I think that if you want to be at an academic program in Boston, by all means you should apply," she said. "Realistically, Brigham, Mass General, and Beth Israel are going to be very difficult. Tufts and Boston University are also difficult, so if your heart is set on Boston you might want to consider some of the secondary affiliates of those medical schools. Have you looked at St. Elizabeth's, Mt. Auburn, Newton-Wellesley, and the Leahy Clinic?"

I indicated that I had not yet really thought about them.

"Well, they would be a good backup plan. If you are set on academic medicine, then you might want to think about expanding your search to the Midwest, or perhaps include other cities on the east coast. That way you will have some options."

So, as I begin my final rotation of my third year, I'm beginning to formulate a plan, and the plan is simply this: Pray that I'm more competitive than everyone takes me to be right now, and apply practically everywhere from Boston to Chicago.

Monday, April 30

The karma of the year had to catch up to me eventually. I've been counting my blessings the entire way through, pleased that I got such cushy schedules as Christ/VA for surgery (when others had the 14- and 15-hour days at the University), and inpatient rotations during the first month of Peds and Medicine, allowing me to study for the all-important tests during the low-impact outpatient second month.

The payback is that for the next two weeks I'll be working labor-and-delivery (or "L & D" as it's shorthanded) at night, trying to figure out how to squeeze in sleep from around 10 a.m. to 5 p.m. In fact, although I'm home right now typing away, I've got to head back to the University and report in at 7 o'clock for my first shift. I was supposed to finish the rest of orientation from three to five, but I figured that it was just another two lectures and I wasn't going to pay much attention to them, so I'm playing hookey before we're even out of the starting gates.

I shouldn't complain; I've got both my weekends off, I'm doing L & D during my first two weeks, and I've got the relatively easy "Continuity of Care" schedule (which apparently corresponds to regular 8-to-5 office hours) during the latter-half of May. But I've been warned that this isn't much consolation. When Aaron Cosgrove, my neighbor and classmate, heard that I was doing nights, he told me, "Steven, I'm not going to sugar-coat this for you. You're fucked. There's no other way to say it delicately."

A lovely sentiment, and that's not the only thing I've heard about this dreaded rotation. The usual medical-student scuttlebutt about various clerkship experiences this year has involved a fairly high degree of variability — this person hated pediatrics, while that person loved it. Different students often have very different takes on the same residents and attendings. That said, I have heard only one person out of at least twenty tell me that they have really enjoyed the OB rotation. At first I thought this might be a gender thing, where the predominantly girls-club atmosphere of the OB/GYN residents was threatening to the male students, who had been totally accustomed to the boys-club atmosphere of the rest of the rotations (with the possible exception of Pediatrics). Not so. One night, Miriam and I had over some friends for drinks, and all but one of the women there concurred that OB was an evil rotation filled largely with evil residents and brutal hours. On the other hand, they said, it's the easiest class to get an "honors" in, so it's not all bad.

Fortunately, I do not have to cope with the most notorious

resident of them all, a chief resident named Jocelyn Gold, who will be working on "MFM," or Maternal and Fetal Medicine. She inspires the same kind of fear and loathing that Joshua Lipschitz does, but because she is a resident, she spends much more time with the students. "The key to surviving Jocelyn Gold," Aaron had said to me when giving me tips on living through the OB rotation, "is to speak only during your patient presentations, and make those very quick and to-the-point. The rest of the time just smile and let her talk, because she doesn't want to hear what you have to say."

Among the stories that have been attributed to her are that she once explained to a retinue of medical students how stupid her patient was while the door to the exam room was wide-open and the patient was easily within earshot, and that she once wrote on the evaluation of an Acting Intern that she couldn't believe that this student wanted to go into OB/GYN, and would be a horrible resident. How much of these details are perfectly accurate is an open question, but as with Lipschitz the amount of bad press indicates that it can't all be the gossip of overly-touchy students who feel maltreated. As I said, though, she's not my problem; my friends Victor and Andrea have to worry about her, as they do MFM during their second two weeks.

ᄋᄋᄋᄋᄋᄋᄋᄋᄋ

I'm one rotation away from being finished with my third year, and it *feels* like I'm moving to a higher level in terms of my training and responsibilities. This is a very different feeling than I had at the end of second year or first year, when one essentially spends time placing one's brain before a book and begs it to soak up as much as possible. One does actually learn incrementally during the first two years but it's hard to be aware of it, simply because the first two years are lived in an educational vacuum — the theme is you versus the test, and you sing that tune over and over again until you take the boards.

But I can look back to who I was ten months ago, when I thought that if I didn't handle a stethoscope right it just might bite me, and I can see that I am, forgive the obviousness of this statement, almost a doctor. During the first few months, when I came in and introduced myself as "student doctor Hatch," I wondered whom I was kidding more, the patients or me. Now I say it because increasingly it makes sense to say so. I'm aware that there's a whole long way to go in terms of how much I need to learn, and that in the spectrum of medical knowledge I'm still a lot closer to the "knows nothing" than the "knows everything" end. But when I started Surgery almost a year ago I felt like I was staring into the void; now the outlines are coming into relief, and the dimly-lit cavern that is "patient care" is becoming brighter daily.

To say that the third-year involves a steep learning curve is an understatement, for it's essentially vertical. You can measure your increase in competency from one *day* to the next, sometimes in hours. When I worked my first night at the newborn nursery I didn't even know how to *hold* a baby, and by the second night I could do a full exam and feel relatively confident that I wasn't making any gross errors. It takes years to build a master clinician, yet it only takes about a year to train someone in the most basic competencies.

For perhaps the first time in my life, I feel like I've become proficient at some tangible thing; I've acquired a set of skills and a way of thinking about the world that will make a real difference in people's lives. I feel like fortune has, if not smiled upon me, then at least winked my way. I suspect that my classmates feel similarly as we wrap up the third year. The overwhelming majority of us are bound for careers in which our hard work will be rewarded with lucrative incomes and a sense of accomplishment. The irony of this feeling is that we have built this good fortune by climbing a heap of discarded limbs, gangrenous toes, ascitic bellies, bleeding rectums, failed hearts and demented brains. We may be in the business to assist our patients, but we nevertheless have attained our success by witnessing their sufferings.

Wednesday, May 2

Has my day started or finished? Hard to tell at this point. Came on at seven last night, worked pretty hard up until about 2:30, then slept until roughly 5:30, but didn't sleep quality hours. Came home and was in bed by 9:30, but my cats refused to let me get more than one consecutive hour of sleep without interruption, so I finally ceded to them by three. I'm on tonight from 7 to 11 p.m., since tomorrow I have lecture from 1 to 5 — but then I have to work later that night from 9 p.m. to 9 a.m. So, in effect, my internal clock is mush.

Still, at least for the moment, I'm not complaining. I'm not complaining because I have almost every weekend off, because after I finish nights L & D I have the cushy 8-to-5 clinic schedule instead of the much more rigorous 5-to-8 MFM schedule, and because I don't have to work with Jocelyn Gold. I haven't heard any new stories about her, but the look of absolute horror in the eyes of Andrea and Jen Alvarez during morning rounds has sufficed. Andrea came up to me after rounds on Tuesday and whispered, "I don't say this very often, but she's the 'C' word."

♀♀♀♀♀♀♀♀♀

Delivered my first baby last night. There is a popular saying in medicine that underlines how medical apprentices obtain their experience: "See one, do one, teach one." I seem to have skipped the "see one" phase for delivering babies, because the only other delivery at which I was in attendance was my own, and my recollections of that event are sufficiently hazy that it wasn't of much help to me in this circumstance.

Mom was a 17 year-old black female and was—so the nurses and residents tell me—one of the happiest women they have ever seen in labor. Since I have seen only one woman in labor, I will take their word for it, although even I could sense that this was an unusually smooth delivery. Mom never once screamed, and in fact managed to *smile* in-between contractions and pushes. The father was probably in the worst shape, since he started getting dizzy and pale and had to lie down through the last ten minutes of labor.

I could tell you about the "cardinal movements of labor" and give you a technical blow-by-blow the way the books describe it, but the truth is that, in the moment, I only consciously understood about three of the movements I was performing: Twist the baby's head from the back to the side once it's out, pull its back shoulder out, and pull its front shoulder out. Everything else happened so fast, and my body was shouting *ADRENALINE! MORE ADRENALINE!* so loudly I could scarcely hear Carol, my intern, walk me through the procedure.

Once the baby's head was out it couldn't have been more than a minute until she was completely out, and lots of maneuvers were happening in the interim. Before I knew it, I was holding this baby with my left hand wrapped around her neck to prevent her from falling (more on this anon) and my right hand supporting baby's body. Then I clamped the cord, Carol cut it, and I zipped the baby over to the pediatric docs for a quick initial evaluation.

If I learned only one lesson, it was this: Babies are slippery. On the first day, during orientation, the course director, Dr. Hopple, had made one or two jokes about making sure *not* to drop the babies when we delivered them. I thought *what?* to myself, thinking it an odd thing to say at the time. I no longer think it's odd.

Given our slippery latex gloves grasping onto a very slimy, wet surface, I wondered to myself just how often people really *did* drop babies. I don't know the answer to that question, but got a rough idea when talking with my best friend Mark earlier today. Mark is a lawyer, and his specialty involves working with hospitals. One thing his firm always does when researching a hospital's financial viability is to learn how many lawsuits against them are pending, including lawsuits involving dropped babies. Which means that as a phenomenon it's common enough to merit its own special designation.

Wednesday, May 9

This morning, as we were rounding on the patients, one of the first-year residents working L&D days named CF was walking behind my second-year resident Amanda. I was asking her a question when I heard a *smack!* from somewhere, and Amanda twisted around immediately.

"CF, *don't* do that." Firm and unambiguous. Amanda is somewhere in her thirties and comes from Armenia via medical school in Romania, while CF looks like a straight-shot to medical school from undergrad, making him about 26, and he looks even younger than that.*

"Do what?" was CF's innocent reply.

"Hit me on my *dupa*," she said. I don't know whether *dupa* is Romanian or Armenian but it was pretty clear what body part *dupa* referred to. "Do not *ever* hit me on the *dupa*."

"But I like hitting you on your *dupa*," said CF, playing along like this was a joke.

There were four medical students there, including two women, Dayva and Charlotte, as well as super-sensitive new-age guy Victor and me. We all looked at each other like we weren't quite sure that what we saw happen actually happened, just because of the sheer preposterousness of the act. "Ummm, CF?" I said. "Do you know how to say, 'sexual harassment'?"

"*That's* not sexual harassment," he said. "She's married! It doesn't count if you're married," he added with a smirk.

I thought, oh dear, he's in for a long residency.

♀♀♀♀♀♀♀♀♀

Since we're on the subject of psychopaths, let's do Horror Stories About Jocelyn Gold, Round Two. I picked up this little ditty at 3 a.m. on Tuesday morning from one of the ER residents named Joanne who did a one-month rotation with the OB team, and had now returned to working the ER. This story involves one of my favorite classmates, George Belron.

---

* I found out later that night that he clocks in at a mere twenty-*four*.

George is one of the smartest and best of our medical students, and I have little doubt that he has been sailing through the year with excellent evaluations.

George had apparently been doing quite well during the OB rotation (which is little surprise), and had earned the respect and trust of everyone on the team. One morning during rounds at the end of George's rotation, Jocelyn was presenting a patient to the attending, and while recalling all of the patient's pertinent info (i.e. her age, her medical history, all of her labs), managed to forget one small little detail. When you deal with dozens of patients on a daily basis, it's very easy to forget one little lab value, so it wasn't a big deal to not be able to recall that information. George, who had been following the patient, called out the value so that the attending knew the number.

One of the cardinal rules for third-year medical students is *never* make your residents look bad. It's important for you to understand that George was *not* doing this. Making your resident look bad means *correcting* them as they're giving a presentation, or supplying information that they have omitted. By contrast, this little moment should have been so trivial that nobody should even have a story to tell. Jocelyn forgot the number (which is no big deal) and George supplied it (which is what a competent student who cares about patient welfare does). The team then had the information and could move on. Jocelyn, however, was so offended by George's "indiscretion" that she rewarded his concern with low-pass marks and a scathing evaluation.

What's to conclude from this story? That, in certain cases, no matter what you do, even if it's the right thing, you're still going to get dinged because you're at the mercy of people much smaller than you. That, if you have the misfortune of running into two or three of these people during your third-year, it could in theory affect your final evaluations and hamper your ability to get into your top-choice programs.

And finally, that I'm in for a very *long* two weeks at the end of my rotation, since I've recently learned that I'm doing gyn surg at Christ hospital with none other than Jocelyn Gold. Apparently I counted my chickens before they were hatched —

such an appropriate metaphor for me—when I said that she wasn't my problem. Then again, it's only fitting that I end the third year the way I started it, among people who need to spend concentrated time with psychiatrists, preferably in lock-down.

♀♀♀♀♀♀♀♀♀

My own experience with the OB residents hasn't been quite as nasty, although of course I haven't gotten an evaluation yet. It also hasn't been the most pleasant of experiences either. One simple problem is due to the vagaries of the calendar, which resulted in a new team coming halfway through our L & D experience. As a consequence, the new team came in with a different set of expectations of what we should know and what we should do. Since the outgoing team was on their eighth week of nights, they weren't very interested in breaking us in, and didn't explain to us how we could do some simple housekeeping-paperwork to help the team function better. The new team came in, and we got three days of, 'You don't know what to write on the discharge summary? Didn't they tell you *anything?* I'm *sure* that you received this information in the packet they give you at orientation.' (We did not.) Once we got a crash-course on paperwork, things have moved a little more smoothly. Of course, we only have 1.5 more nights left with the team, so it's a little late to make much of a difference.

I work mainly with two residents, one of whom I like, the other of whom I don't. Amanda (the resident I mentioned above) and I were off to a good start together the moment I started working with her. When she told me she was from Romania, I asked her if she was there while Caeucescu was in power. She was so blown away that an American had even *heard* of Caeucescu that she couldn't stop talking about it for the next half-hour, and I knew that I had made an impression, even if it had no bearing on obstetrics and gynecology.

Lucy Imani is the first-year resident, a five-foot-four lady with an engagement ring that weighs in at three carats and who insists on wearing full makeup to night call. While I won't put her on my "ten most admired residents of third year" list, she could be a lot worse. She reminds me faintly of Jenny Wang, who was torture to be around on a personal level, but generally is professional and takes the time to teach when something of medical consequence happens.

That said, I had a rather unpleasant incident with her this morning. We had a long night, having admitted several patients to L & D as well as a patient from the ER for suspected endomyometritis — an infection of the uterus that can occur after Cesearean section delivery. Lucy wanted me to follow that woman and present her in the morning rounds. I had to visit the patients that had given birth yesterday in addition to that, which wasn't much of a big deal and took 45 minutes tops.

The problem came when Amanda and I saw a woman in triage who had just gone into labor at about 4:00 a.m. At first, it looked like it was going to be a long labor, but by five it was clear that she was going to deliver sometime that morning. I very much wanted to be at the delivery since I was only going to be on L & D for two weeks of my entire professional life, and thus far I had only delivered one baby. The problem was as we approached 5:30, I knew that Lucy was expecting me to round on the routine post-partum patients as well as our ER admit. I asked Amanda what to do. "Here's the thing," I said. "The residents have to write their own notes anyway, so it's not like I'm doing anything critical up there. And I'm not learning anything *new* by interviewing my tenth post-partum patient. But on the other hand, I'm not going to get too many more chances to be at a delivery, and *that's* what I'm here for, right?"

"Yeah, I agree with you," she said. "It's your call, but you might want to check it out, or quickly write some notes and get back here, so that you don't get in any trouble."

So, off I dashed to the wards, quickly interviewed two moms and sketched off two notes. I didn't see Lucy around so I was going to head up to the 8th floor to talk to the woman with the endomyometrial infection. By this point, all of the students had come in to round and were writing notes in the nursing station.

Just then Lucy came steaming through. She looks right at me: "Steven, I didn't see your note on Ms. Broderick!" First thing out of her mouth, loud enough so that everyone in the room could hear.

I turned just a lighter shade than purple. "*Well*," I replied, "I just *happened* to finish writing my notes on the patients on *this* floor first, and before that I came from L & D where a mom is delivering as we speak, so it's not like I've been dallying. I was on my way up there right now." I think my other classmates saw that I was prepared to pull her tongue out.

"Oh," was her nonchalant reply, and she went about her business.

I went up to interview Ms. Broderick, who was in so foul a mood that the Chief Resident for the daytime shift, Tony, told me not to bother with her and that he'd handle it, up to and including presenting her at rounds. With that, I decided to head back to the delivery room. It was 6:30 a.m., and she had delivered about twenty minutes earlier. Amanda was completing the repair of an episiotomy, when she looked up at me and said, "You couldn't get away, could you?"

Thursday, May 10

At the beginning of the shift last night, one of the senior residents was working on a case that classmate Dara and I were explicitly instructed *not* to attend. Normally I would assume this to be a private patient, but private patients typically don't want resident coverage, either. They want to deal only with the attending, and that's that.

Later in the night, I found out from Amanda what happened, after Jennifer, the senior resident, had debriefed the other residents. "Jen said it was pretty awful. Some woman came in about twenty-four weeks with a septic abortion. Someone had done a back-alley job and made a terrible mess of it. Jen had her hands in there, pulling out the baby's body parts, and it was green and smelled terribly foul, I guess."

"Jesus!" I said. "Why didn't she just get an abortion from

a clinic a few months ago?" Abortions are legal and available in this country — so far, anyway — through the first trimester. After that, there are only a few places that will perform safe abortions, but even then no one will mess with a pregnancy after about the 22nd week. No one reputable, anyway. A "septic" abortion means an abortion that causes a systemic infection and, if not treated, is lethal.

"Beats me. You know, I used to see this all the time."

"You did?"

"Yeah, in medical school in Romania. When I lived in Romania, it was illegal to get an abortion, punishable by death. So women would roll in to the hospital in sepsis all the time. But here's the best part: The police would find out about the women, and they wouldn't allow us to treat them until they gave up the name of the person who performed the abortion. So we'd see women die all the time, refusing to implicate anyone. Yeah, everyone's talking about this being so unusual. This was bread-and-butter in my medical school."

If you do not think fundamentalist Christians are the enemy, take note.

♀♀♀♀♀♀♀♀♀

An obstetrics resident's view of the world:

"Um, Amanda?"

"Yeah, Steven, what's up?"

"Did you see Shamiqua's eye on exam?" I ask her this just before we start rounds at seven. Shamiqua, an eighteen year-old, had just given birth to her second baby boy.

"No, I didn't. Why?"

"Because she had what looked like a small hemorrhage in her sclera, maybe a couple of millimeters wide. I made a note about it."

"Steven, if it's not inside the box, then I don't worry about it." The "box" being the region starting at the vulva, going out to the ovaries, and finishing at the fundus of the uterus.

Friday, May 11

On my final night of L&D, I got tapped on the shoulder at 3:30 by Amanda, who said that someone was cooking down in the ER and we had been consulted. On the way down, Amanda waxed eloquent about her hatred of the ER residents. Now, at the end of my third year, I've learned a lesson that I would scarcely have believed true at the beginning: Nearly everyone hates ER residents. Surgery residents, Medicine residents, now OB residents. The main problem focuses on "turfing," the process by which an ER doc delegates responsibility of the care of a patient to a different medical or surgical specialty. A patient comes in with bad belly pain suggestive of appendicitis? They most likely go to a surgery resident. Someone comes in with confusion, lethargy, and vomiting? Call the medicine or neuro residents pronto.

Although I've never talked to ER residents about it, my guess is that from their perspective they need to move patients quickly, and when they see a patient that can be adequately managed by another specialty, then they call them in. It's such an ingrained mentality that their underground motto, "Surf 'em and turf 'em," has been uttered more than once on the show *ER*. The complaint from the other docs is that they turf cases that they should, in theory, be able to handle adequately on their own.

"Steven," Amanda said, waving a finger, "their residents come up to work with us for a month or two, and *the whole point* is to give them some basic training so that they don't consult us every time they get a positive beta," referring to the pregnancy test. "I mean, do I really need to come down and spend forty-five minutes, an hour, or more, to leave the work I'm needed to do upstairs, to do all that paperwork *just* so that I can tell them that someone's got a normal pregnancy? This is ridiculous!"

The patient we came to see down in the ER, however, was *not* "just" a positive beta. This woman, Vanessa Artest, had left the hospital AMA (against medical advice) two days ago. We got down to the ER and tracked down the resident to get the story, who grimaced when we mentioned her name. "Oh she's

in sixteen," she said. "Watch out for her. She's got one very
nasty temper."

"Why did she leave? What was she here for?" Amanda
asked.

"Beats me *why*," the resident said. "She's got endometritis,
and she doesn't look good."

She wasn't kidding. Endometritis, or "endomyometritis"
as it's officially called, is a moderately serious condition that
occurs in mothers who have had a recent C-section. The lining
of the uterus (the endometrium) along with the musculature
of the uterus (the myometrium) become infected, often with
multiple organisms, and usually within a week of giving birth
mom gets sick. The treatment is to pound the patient with
antibiotics and give them rest. Like all internal infections, the
consequences of not treating it are, at best, severe, and at worst
fatal.

Leaving AMA without having finished treatment was very,
very risky, and now she had returned less than 48 hours later,
and looked terrible. Before we even stepped into the room to
talk to her, we looked over the ER admission sheet, and saw
her vitals, showing a temperature of 104°, a heart rate of 130
(high-normal is 100), and a low-normal blood pressure. We
could *hear* her moaning, standing twenty feet away, and the
ER is a very noisy place. Amanda was already angry about the
whole situation. "What is the matter with this woman?" she
asked as she read over the history. "Why do people do such
stupid things to themselves and then expect *us* to make things
better?"

My guess at that point was that crack could give someone
a craving that bad that they'd leave the hospital to get high.
Based on what I had seen, it was a good guess, but it wouldn't
prove to be right.

We came in and saw an 18 year-old girl in shorts, a t-shirt
that covered half her belly, and a Knicks cap on. She was pulled
up in a ball on the gurney and looked very uncomfortable.
When we introduced ourselves, she said, "What the fuck is
going on? Can't you guys give me something so that I can get
out of here?"

"No, we can't do that—"

"Well, why the fuck not—"

"Because you're very sick, and we're going to need to admit you."

"No fuckin' way! Listen, gimme somethin' cuz I'm getting the fuck outta here."

Amanda took a deep breath. "Ms. Artest, do you know what's wrong with you? Do you know that you're going to *die* if you leave before we can treat you properly? It's going to take us *days* to get you better. Do you want your baby to lose her mother at one week old?"

That seemed to work the magic, and suddenly this nasty ball of rage started sobbing hysterically. "I just want my baby," she kept saying over and over. Amanda turned to me and asked if she could have some time alone with her, and would I please check some labs.

About five minutes later, Amanda emerged, looking like she had just been through war, which in a way she had. It turned out she had *two* kids, the second child a two year-old, and the children were the source of the problem, not crack cocaine. However, crack played a starring role in the whole tangled drama. Ms. Artest, all of eighteen, left the hospital because she didn't trust her mother, who *was* a crack addict, to watch over her two children. She had no other friends on whom she could rely. None. This obviously left her in a pickle: Care for herself and put her children at risk, or watch over her children and risk grave illness.

Amanda shook her head, and looked to me for any thoughts. Fortunately I had one. "Why don't we talk to the social workers?" I said. Social workers, I have come to believe, can be a very useful ally. The problem with them is that the variability in skill level is even wider than that of nurses and doctors, the good ones being priceless and the bad ones being detrimental to the patients' welfare. There are ways of getting around bad nurses, bad residents, and bad attendings; but a social worker has a set of skills and a knowledge base that the medical folk simply don't possess, so once you call them in, minimizing their impact is difficult.

Fortunately, the social workers in this case came to talk to Ms. Artest and then came to us before asking if they should proceed, which was wise since the news wasn't very good. They said they could call in Social Services, a branch of the county government, who could watch over the kids, take them into their custody, until she had recovered. That was a risky strategy, though. "You see, if Social Services takes the kids, they're going to investigate the case, and an 18 year-old woman with no social support to watch over her kids, no job, no ability to *hold* a job because of the problem with child care.... well, it's quite possible she could lose custody of the children altogether. Do you want us to call them?"

"No," was the immediate and simultaneous response that Amanda and I gave, and we were back to square one. It was pushing five at this point, and we were going to be needed upstairs to round on the post-partum moms in less than a half hour. Amanda looked at me with tired eyes and said she had an idea.

"I don't know what else to do," she said. "I'm going to call the mom and try and get the two of them together and have an understanding that she's got to watch over these kids for the next week. She can't go out again. This is my best thought at the moment."

We negotiated between the mother and the daughter for all of the 25 minutes that we had before we had to bug out. As we let it stand, Vanessa agreed to stay in the hospital for at least three days while we got her the necessary IV medications. She needs at least seven days of antibiotics, but we're going to have to settle for what we can get with her. I suggested that we try to get her a 'PICC' line, a device which would allow us to give her IV medications as an outpatient. It's a device normally reserved for patients who need two or three *months* of IV antibiotics, like those with osteomyelitis or endocarditis (infections involving the bone and the inside lining of the heart), but given the possible catastrophic consequences of her leaving again I figured it was worth a shot to at least look into it. It would require some administrative tap-dancing, though. That, however, will be someone else's problem.

Mother swore that she'd watch after the kids.

We finished up our note and headed up to Three, so that I could do the last post-partum rounds, and changing of the board, of my entire, grateful, life.

♀♀♀♀♀♀♀♀♀

As you'll recall, during my rotation in General Surgery I expressed my love for really bloody surgeries — after all, a good surgery needs blood squishing and sloshing all over the place, right? Well, general surgery's got *nothing* on Obstetrics. During my two-week stint on L & D, I attended about four C-sections, and it's simply incredible how much blood is lost during this procedure. My residents guessed that the typical blood loss is about a liter or more (it's considerably less in a vaginal delivery). So, budding surgeons take note: If you want to go into a field where you'll get your hands *red*, there's no question that OB/GYN is your game.

Wednesday, May 16

The patients in University Hospital's OB ward are, by and large, very different from other patients that I have been dealing with throughout the year. I got used to seeing two types of patients as the year progressed: One kind were the VA patients, mostly hard-working, hard-drinking, heavy-smoking proles who, despite being in miserable health, had pleasant dispositions; the other were insured private-practice outpatients that held down jobs of varying degrees of income and responsibility and usually came to the office for help with non-devastating medical problems. They took exactly the opposite approach of the Vets toward the health care system: They came to doctors before their problems had ruined them.

The only time I had encountered patients at the true bottom of the social and economic scale was when I worked on psychiatry, and even then it was difficult to visualize how they functioned in their native environment, since they were so far-removed in the confines of the lock-down ward or the drug-rehab house. When I went to the jail and worked in the psych emergency room, though, I got a whiff, sometimes literally, of where they came from, and I appreciated in a new way just how sheltered my comfortable life is.

Many of the young women who come walking through the door to the OB triage have much in common with those psych patients in that they are often coming from the same kind of environment, which isn't particularly nurturing, especially to unwed teenage mothers of multiple children. At the University Hospital, this kind of mom is the rule rather than the exception, and I believe that it contributes in part to the overall low morale of the OB residents. Every night they are confronted on multiple occasions with an America so wholly different from the Gingerbread-House-In-The-Suburbs variety that it sometimes seems they view these women as opponents in a war of attrition rather than patients requiring the gentle, smooth touch of a caretaker.

After the third or fourth night I came to, if not empathize, then at least understand the feelings of the residents. Easily, 60 percent of the women who come in through the OB triage door each night are teenagers, are on their second, third, or fourth pregnancy, are lucky if they have one or two years of high-school education, and have little or no prospects for a job with any kind of meaningful income or health insurance anywhere on the horizon.

These women are also frequently infected with various sexually-transmitted diseases such as chlamydia and gonorrhea (from male partners who often refused or ignored treatment, causing a continuous reinfection cycle). Sometimes they are the victims of sexual abuse and other times "just" physical abuse. The prenatal care that they got came not through regular appointments in a clinic provided by the hospital, but rather from obstetric triage, where they came whenever they felt the need. It didn't take long to hear a niggling question in the back of my head that no doubt has flashed through the mind of every half-alert resident here: *How on earth can a kid be raised by a mother like this in an environment like that?*

One of the first of these women I saw, Cara, was a 22 year-old from a small town called Maysville, Kentucky, a town of only 10,000 people about an hour from Cincinnati. She had been treated there for most of her pregnancy, but came to live with a friend in a Cincinnati neighborhood on the west side of town for reasons about which she remained vague. She was in her seventh month and was complaining of contractions. This was Cara's sixth pregnancy, and she had four living children. She was educated through 8th grade. She came in with her friend to see what we could do about the contractions, which she was having maybe once every ten minutes. Her water hadn't broke and she wasn't bleeding. Since there was nothing obviously acutely wrong with her, this struck me as somewhat odd. It was three o'clock in the morning; at that point she could have just waited a few more hours and tried to schedule a same-day appointment at the clinic.

As I was trying to get a medical history from Cara, her friend—wearing a spaghetti-strap shirt that left most of her belly and the entirety of her back exposed, tight-fitting jeans, and yes, *makeup* at 3 a.m.—was shouting at someone at the receiving end of a call from her cell phone, apparently regarding who was going to watch over *her* children while she was tending to her friend. "Goddamn it, you fuckin' bitch," she said at a volume sufficiently loud that it could be heard well down the hallway through a closed door. "All's I do is watch over *yer* kids and you can't help me out this time! We'll *see* if I *ever* help your fuckin' ass out of a problem ever again!" Pause. "Fuck you, too!"

Despite all the best social graces I could muster, I clearly looked bewildered and Cara knew it.

"Darlene?" asked Cara. "Could you quiet down a little? The doctor can't hear me."

Darlene wheeled around at us in total surprise, like perhaps *we* had interrupted *her*. "Oh," she said, wide-eyed. "Sorry about that."

Then she turned quickly to the phone, said, "You know what, fuck you. Just fuck you," and promptly hung up.

It got worse. When I finally obtained Cara's limited medical records I saw something funny about having been diagnosed with cervical cancer *five years ago* but not yet having received treatment. Cervical cancer is believed to be exclusively caused by a sexually-transmitted virus, the human papilloma virus. Pap smears check for changes that papilloma virus can cause, and she had a few abnormal paps several years back, but hadn't done anything about them.

"Hey, Amanda, take a look at this note," I said as I pointed out the information on the pap smears and "cervical cancer." The note from the Maysville hospital didn't make it clear whether the patient or the doctor was reporting it as cancer. If it was the patient, it was somewhat less worrisome, because Cara may have been warned that, if untreated, her abnormal paps would eventually *lead* to cancer, and then Cara misunderstood this as a diagnosis *of* cancer and reported it as such. If it was the doctor reporting it as cancer, however, it was much less likely to be such an innocent error, in which case she had full-fledged, untreated cervical cancer, and depending on how long she waited for treatment, she was in grave danger. If she persisted in opting for no treatment, regardless of the stage of cancer or of "dysplasia" — the pre-cancerous state picked up by the pap smears — she was going to die from cervical cancer.

When Amanda came to see Cara, it wasn't a happy encounter. "Look, do you want to die?" Amanda asked. "This is a disease that we can prevent one-hundred percent, but you've got to do your part and get treatment for it. Do you want to have your kids grow up without a mother?"

Cara looked at her with a mix of slack-jawed terror and annoyance that Amanda was being so rude to her at this visit. "Ummm...."

"...because that's what's going to happen to you if you don't do something about this now," Amanda continued. "You're going to die. It's that simple."

We ended up sending her home that night — she wasn't in labor, and there wasn't anything further we could do for her except refer her to the clinic to arrange for follow-up on the dysplasia/cancer that she may have had for quite a while.

Cara wasn't even the best representative sample. We'd see a 16 year-old who was on her second pregnancy and coming in at 33 weeks because she too thought she might be in labor. This was her first visit for *any* kind of prenatal care. She knew that there was a clinic where she could be seen by the residents, and she had made a few appointments, but she couldn't keep them because she was "too busy." We'd see a 17 year-old who kept coming in with chlamydia because her partner wasn't going in for treatment; the woman/girl would keep shouting at her three year-old to shut-the-fuck-up for whining about being in a hospital at two in the morning. Then we'd see a 15 year-old who was having her first child but no father was anywhere in sight. And so on.

With the vast majority of these women, you wouldn't see *anything* that could be regarded as a good omen for the future: No source of income, little or no social support network, no education, no apparent sign of being tied to a religious or spiritual group that might provide some kind of help. These girls had apparently received no training in how to deal with life's stresses, like raising a kid in the world on the bottom rung of the social ladder, alone, with no assistance.

My first gut reaction was largely of disgust. Several of the residents were less shy about their feelings, which were similar but much more engrained by that point. They'd often walk briskly into these patients rooms and do all of the things that we are repeatedly told not to do to patients—not make eye contact, ask questions in a cold manner, cut off patient responses—just to minimize the amount of time they had to deal with such patients. The patients were keenly aware of the negative vibe in the room and often responded with hostility in kind. The ice-breakers, if they occurred, would come when we had to do a sonogram or strap on the tocolytic and fetal-heart monitors. When the focus changed to the baby, everyone got more pleasant, at least marginally so.

I've been around many patients who have histories totally alien to mine. They aren't college or high-school educated, come from low social classes, and almost go out of their way to not take care of themselves. However, if they were pleasant—and the Vets were especially pleasant—I didn't think of the encounter as anything fundamentally different than dealing with a well-educated suburbanite except for how I tried to explain the medical plan.

By contrast, I saw so much nastiness in the OB triage between the patient and the mother, between the patient and her child, between the patient and the baby's father, or any combination of these people. I couldn't understand what caused people to be so mean, and after a while all *I* wanted to do was get out of those rooms.

When you spend time observing these situations, watching people in bad circumstances make bad decisions, you see a bleak future but are powerless to stop it. Many of these young women aren't taking care of themselves, and at least some of them will have children who will become Someone Else's Problem in fifteen or twenty years when they are involved in drugs, prostitution, violent crime, or are having children themselves that they cannot support financially. That means that taxpayers will be footing the bill. I've felt outraged watching these mothers who are receiving *free* care and are totally ungrateful about it. After seeing this happen three times a night, every night, for two weeks, I began to think that maybe Republicans have a point.

I very much doubt I'd actually vote for a Republican unless it was one seriously liberal dude, but I'm not sure how I'd feel after four years of being relentlessly pounded with patients like these that are seen every day by the residents on the University OB service. That kind of brutal assault on the senses no doubt hardens them, and I can't blame them for their bitterness and oft-stated desire to have a job working in the burbs.

Wednesday, May 23

The Continuity Of Care clinic represents an age-old solution to the dilemma of how apprentice doctors gain experience. After all, most patients don't want to be "practiced upon" by fresh graduates of medical schools who have not yet learned enough to be competent on their own. But *somebody* has to be the patient-base for young doctors, else there would be no new doctors to fill the ranks. Thus, most residency programs in the country serve patients who can't have the option of choosing a doctor — that is, poor people. And Vets.

The COC clinic is therefore one of the major inner-city gynecology clinics in Cincinnati. The overwhelming majority of patients are black or Appalachian, in contrast to the overwhelming majority of obstetric residents, who are white suburbanites. Many of the residents appear to enjoy their clinic time since they get to "take possession" of their patients, having direct responsibility for their care during the four years of their residency.

But there are also many residents who harbor a great deal of resentment toward several of their patients, especially those that will not take care of themselves or their children. And there's often *many* children, children being supervised by mothers who aren't far out of childhood themselves and totally unprepared for the financial and physical demands of motherhood. Even after only a week of COC, despite all my good pinko-faggot-liberal leanings, I can easily sympathize with the frustrations of the residents. After all, how many times do you have to hear the phrase "shut the fuck up" during a routine office visit before you think that's just an expression of affection between a mother and her three year-old?

Today, though, I saw two patients who didn't fit this mold. The first was Laetitia Cassocks, and on her chart was written "appointment for permanent sterilization," meaning that this was a pre-op evaluation for a tubal ligation, where the fallopian tubes are cauterized and sealed so that eggs may not travel from the ovaries to the uterus. My resident, Helen, who was completing her final month of residency, told me to go into the room, get the basic story, and report back to her. As I entered, I saw a young black woman with two children, one about three, the other an infant.

"Hi there," I said as gently as possible, and introduced myself and explained my mission. She explained that she was a single mother, age 20, trying to raise these kids, work full time, and take college classes one-by-one working toward an associate degree. Her mother and some other family helped out with the kids. She had a working plan of how to make things better, but she was obviously overwhelmed by the responsibility that came with having two children before finishing her teens.

As we talked I realized that I didn't like the idea of her sterilization at all. Twenty years old and with *six* kids, or just twenty years old and stupid? I had no problem with that kind of a situation. But this girl was obviously bright, and she had a very long reproductive life ahead of her. What would happen, I thought, if she does get that college degree, gets herself on firm financial footing by the time she's thirty, then meets a guy who wants to get married and have kids? Can she be certain now, with all of the wisdom that comes at age 20, that she won't *ever* want to have another child?

Granted, it wasn't my decision to make. She's the patient, and it's her choice (unless the doctors refuse to perform the procedure). But there are ways to sell a medical or surgical plan to a patient, particularly one with limited understanding of all the options for contraception. I asked her why she wouldn't take oral contraceptive pills. She said that she just forgot to take the pill too often—which is how she ended up with the second child. And condoms, given the reluctance of her partners, were strictly out of the question.

"That's fine," I said, though I was disappointed by her inability to figure out a way of taking a little pill every morning—like, how hard is it to put it by your toothbrush and take one every morning when you hit the bathroom? But I had another thought. "Have you ever heard of an IUD?" I asked.

She hadn't. If I have learned something during this rotation (and I have learned precious little, my attitude being as poor as it is as we race across the finish line of the third year), it is that the Intra-Uterine Device is a woefully underused tool in contraception. A relatively tiny copper-and-plastic "T", sometimes laced with progesterone, the IUD is inserted directly into the patient's uterus right there in the exam room, and can provide protection at about the same rate as the pill (which is very close to 100 percent) for *up to ten years*! And unlike pills, which are pretty safe in their own right, there are even fewer side effects with IUDs.

Unfortunately, IUDs have had a terribly bad rap in this country due to a fiasco with one particular brand of IUD, the Dalkon Shield, which caused a great deal of trouble with women in the mid 1970's. After a host of nasty reactions, up to and including death, the makers of the Dalkon Shield were sued, successfully. The lawsuit generated headlines, and clinical researchers produced studies which purportedly showed that IUDs were not safe forms of contraception. These studies were quite recently shown, in retrospect, to be inaccurate, because if one excluded the patients who had the Dalkon Shield, the *other* IUDs were safe. But by now, more than twenty years later, the general public equates IUD with some unspeakable medical catastrophe.

Thus, for a person who wants to have long-term contraception but not necessarily permanent sterility and who either can't or won't take the pill, an IUD is a perfect solution. It can be taken out whenever the patient wants, so an unplanned desire to have babies isn't impossible to accommodate. In short, an IUD was a fabulous solution for Laetitia Cassocks, who by my reckoning was too young to know what the future might hold and had not yet single-handedly overpopulated the earth.

I spent several minutes explaining how it worked, the advantages it had for her in particular, its safety, and above all its ability to keep her options open. I explained to her that *half* of all women who undergo tubal ligation experience regret at some time following their sterilization. I related that I certainly had no idea at age 20 that I'd be in medical school at age 30 — the future held so much possibility for her, why shut a part of it down?

She smiled at me, but I could see that she didn't even want to *think* about another option. She had made this appointment knowing that she wanted the surgery, and wasn't really going to listen to anything else on the table. My guess is that she arrived at her decision after one long vomit-filled night with one of the children, totally exhausted from her work and the requirements of this infant, who wasn't more than four or five months old. That night, she probably said, "That's it, I'm done.

No more of this ever again." And that's not a good time to make a decision of this magnitude.

I explained that I would go discuss this with the resident, but that I'd *really* like her to consider what I said while I was out, and that the two of us would return in a few minutes. When I hit the resident room I summarized everything that I had just told Laetitia. "Listen, we can't just let her sign that consent," I said.

"Why not?" asked Helen.

"Because I don't think she's doing this with a totally clear mind. I think she's exhausted from the baby, and she's *twenty*, for God's sake, she has *no idea* what the future's gonna bring."

"Do you think she's competent to make the decision? Legally?"

"Yes, but—"

"It sounds like you spent some time explaining the IUD."

"Yes, I did."

"Then it sounds like she's made her decision, and I'm not going to interfere with it."

"Wait, Helen. Can't we at least have her follow up with us, say, in three months? Let's give her some time to mull over the IUD. She's so hot to get to the operating room that she's not listening to anything else. If she wants to get consented in three months, fine. But why the rush?"

Helen looks at me carefully. She's the kind of resident you like to work with as a medical student, not only because she's pleasant, but because she actually takes the time to listen to you and give you feedback. Many of the OB residents in clinic wouldn't even deign to have this conversation. "Steven, there's something you have to understand. You're here for two weeks. I've been here four years, and I can't tell you the number of times that I've seen women that I'd *love* to sterilize—women with four, five, six kids, who don't know what they're doing, and we're going to end up seeing *their* kids in the clinic in about fifteen years. So when someone comes along and *wants* a tubal, I don't ask many questions. I make sure they know the risks so they can make an informed decision, but all I'm thinking is: Sign on the dotted line."

Less than ten minutes later, Laetitia Cassocks signed the consent form.

♀♀♀♀♀♀♀♀♀

"Helen, you're not going to believe this," I said as I came into the residents' office later that day.

Chase Furlow didn't look like a typical COC patient at all, and she was obviously a new patient since her chart was essentially empty. As with Ms. Cassocks, a big post-it note was placed on the front of the chart, saying that she was here for a tubal consent. When I came in, there were three children sitting with her — all well-groomed and dressed in very nice clothes, as was she. This did not appear to be a woman who needed to be at this clinic. I saw her infant, less than two months old, and asked her how the delivery went.

"Oh, it was fine," she said. "Fourth time around, you know. I delivered at Mercy Anderson." This is one of the smaller, Catholic, private hospitals on the edge of town, with mostly suburban fare walking through its doors.

"Really? Then what brings you here?"

"Because at Mercy they won't even talk to you about contraception."

Catholics. Love those guys. "So, I see you're here because you want a tubal ligation."

"Yes, that's right."

"You're twenty-four?"

"Yes."

"Have you ever heard of an IUD?"

"What's that?"

And so it went. At four children, I realize that she was a less ideal candidate for an IUD than Ms. Cassocks (or rather, less ideal for having an additional child: There's nothing that says she can't have an IUD until she hits menopause), but I still didn't like permanent sterility for someone that young. And as before, Ms. Furlow didn't want to hear about IUDs, she wanted to hear about how soon she could shut down her reproductive machinery.

When I approached Helen, though, the argument was still the same one, and I didn't have much of a response to her logic. Shortly thereafter she signed the consent.[*]

Sunday, May 27

I just spent twenty-four hours of my life on-call at the L & D ward as part of my clerkship requirement. This is my last call for the obstetric portion of the course (I'll take call again next month during gyn surgery at Christ), and it was packed with delieveries, not all of them pleasant. I think I was supposed to learn something about indications for using terbutaline in premature labor, but the real lesson that I learned this weekend was that I have little but naked contempt for those who believe in "natural" childbirth.

Among the many deliveries yesterday was a less pleasant one that involved a woman whom I had seen last week at the COC clinic. We both liked each other at that meeting, and when I saw her come to the hospital in labor I thought it was a special treat for my last day — I get to deliver someone that I've met before and who's comfortable with me. We whisked her from the OB triage area to the delivery suites, which are among the most comfortable rooms in the entire hospital. When we got her situated, she was having contractions about every five or so minutes.

I figured she wouldn't break a sweat. This was a lady in her mid-thirties, and this was her sixth child. Based on what I had been told in lecture and by the residents, multigravids (women who have had many children) have a tendency to deliver

---

[*] I want to point out, for the sake of completeness, that "permanent" sterility is not absolutely permanent. As long as a woman has functional ovaries and a healthy uterus, it is possible for a woman with a tubal to undergo In Vitro Fertilization and become pregnant. However, such procedures don't come cheap, running upwards of $10,000. Chase Furlow *might* be able to afford such an expense several years down the road; it's highly unlikely that Laetitia Cassocks will ever earn enough to afford IVF. When weighed against the almost laughably inexpensive IUD (a few hundred dollars for five to ten years of contraception), banking on an IVF just in case one changes one's mind seems thoroughly foolish.

quickly and without much fuss. In fact, one of the nights I was working L & D we had a woman brought in by the EMTs who had labored so quickly, the baby was delivered even prior to the ambulance arriving.

Nevertheless, it was pretty apparent by the time we had her settled and comfortable that she was not at all happy. "Can you guys get me an epidural?" she asked plaintively. "This is hurting like a bitch!"

"We'll see what we can do," said my resident-du-jour. "We'll give anesthesia a call, and hopefully we'll get them down here as soon as possible."

But, two hours of screaming later, the anesthesia residents were nowhere in sight, and after a breakpoint at the University, moms don't get epidurals if delivery is imminent, which it appeared to be in this case. Mom was *screaming*, and had been in agony for almost the entire time. "I'm *not* going to do this," she kept saying.

"Yes, you are," said my resident. "You've *got* to do this, or else you'll harm your baby."

"Fuck the baby," she replied. "This *hurts!*"

The delivery, without anesthesia, was completed about two hours later, and although mom was delighted with the results, she wasn't very happy in the interim. Why on earth someone would forgo the comfort of an epidural because it's not "natural," and scream and writhe in pain for hours on end, is completely beyond my understanding.

Or *almost* beyond my understanding. I suppose I could be sympathetic to moms who really took the meaning of "natural" the whole way, and didn't want to have any technology associated with their pregnancy—no triple screens, no regular OB visits, no ultrasounds, nothing—because then I'd at least acknowledge their intellectual consistency. They'd be stupid, but they'd at least show that they understand the meaning of the word "natural." But for moms who want to *say* they did it naturally, meaning they did it without an epidural, all I can think is: Why, if you're willing to rely on technology for everything else, would you not let technology help control your *pain*? Does that make the experience better for you?

I was thinking about this specifically in relation to one of the more common complications of pregnancy, the *placenta previa*. Placenta previa occurs when the placenta — the amalgam of tissue that supports the baby throughout pregnancy — sits directly above the cervix, making it impossible, or at least very difficult, for baby to pass through the birth canal without ripping to shreds the very tissue that keeps it alive. The "treatment" for placenta previa, we learned during lecture, is a caesarean section.

In one of my more lucid moments that afternoon, I grabbed one of the course directors, who happened to be in to look after one of his private patients. "Hey," I said. "I was just thinking about your lecture on previas, and I was wondering: How did you diagnose a previa before ultrasounds were around?"

"Oh, it was pretty much a guessing affair," the doc said. "Vaginal bleeding was one of the signs, but of course a lot of things can cause vaginal bleeding during pregnancy. Often they'd make the diagnosis when they would go to deliver the baby, and the doctor or midwife would put his or her hand right through the placenta. Unless they got them out fast, the mother would exsanguinate. The babies were already dead, effectively. The only thought at that point was of saving the mom, but mostly they'd die, too."

Word to you future moms out there: You want natural childbirth, *that's* a natural childbirth. Good luck to you and your ten percent chance of dying, to say nothing of your kid's survival chances.

Tuesday, May 29

Now I'm in the "preceptor" portion of the course — the two-week period devoted to an outpatient office experience with private-practice docs. My private is a mid-forties guy named Santakis. He's a huge man, standing a few inches above me (and I'm a fairly big guy at six-two) with a Thurman Munson walrus-style mustache (or, if you're not a baseball fan, then a 'stache in the manner of David Crosby). He appears to have an equally huge personality: Outgoing, bantering with all his staff

271

(which includes his wife and brother-in-law), openly planning his next baseball outing, and always speaking in an upbeat way. "Bullish" is the word I'd use as my first-impression word. I like him, and I'm pretty sure I'll enjoy the next ten days that I hang out with him.

Santakis is one of the few remnants of a dying breed: An OB doc who is in solo practice. Solo practices are going the way of the dodo in all fields of medicine, but it's especially rare to find one in OB, since being a solo practitioner means that you're on call every hour of every day that you work. If some mom (or rather, some baby) decides that it's time to go at 2:45 a.m. on the far side of town, then he gets the call and he drives over there to deliver the baby. Plus, there's the sticky situation of trying to schedule vacations.

It sounds like he's got privileges at practically all the major hospitals in town, which means that he's got to spend a crushing amount of time just commuting to do his job. He claims that he's got better overhead and, astonishingly, *more* free time now that he's in solo practice after leaving a group practice in Massachusetts, but I'm convinced that, as a matter of pure statistics, he must have had a few nights over the past ten years where he's delivered babies on four or five consecutive nights and gotten practically no sleep. How someone could work that hard is beyond me. But then, I haven't gone through residency yet, and I'll *never* go through a surgery residency, probably the single most brutal medical experience still available for those foolhardy enough to participate.

Just got off the phone with classmate Vikash. He actually worked with Santakis when he did OB. He confirmed my sense that it was going to be a relatively relaxed two weeks and that he was a pretty good character. Still, he had one surprise. "Steve, the guy's a total Republican," he told me.

"Really?"

"Yeah, watch what you say around him about politics. I was working with him right before the election, and everything was about Bush-this and Bush-that. I didn't say much to him when he'd talk to me about that stuff, just tried to make it sound like

I was a centrist and moderate, which I guess I am, except that I can't imagine voting for a Republican."

"Jesus! He's from Massachusetts!"

"Yeah, I know. *Big*-time Republican."

"Well, I guess that he made the right move in coming here to Cincinnati. At least here, he fits in with the prevailing belief system."

"Seriously."

♀♀♀♀♀♀♀♀
♂♂♂♂♂♂♂♂♂

Did I mention that Miriam's pregnant?

Yeah, Miriam's pregnant. I'm convinced it's got something to do with the pheromones of those women on the OB service, because not only are the whopping majority of patients pregnant, but half the nurses and residents are as well. There's something like four or five pregnant residents out of 28 in the UC program. All's I can say is that we've been having trouble for over a year now, and soon as I hit the OB team, boom! Ovulation and Implantation! Coincidence? I think not.

Having Miriam become pregnant right now, while I'm actively tending to pregnant women, is a mixed blessing. You'd think it should be such a wonderful experience to be around such joyous women while I do this rotation, that it should be so encouraging and I should feel such exuberance knowing that I will experience this happiness myself sometime at the end of next January.

Instead, I feel like I'm face-to-face with all of the things that can go *wrong* with a pregnancy and wonder whether or not we'll ever make it to a full-term, nice, normal baby. The odds that she'll even make it to term are somewhere between one-half and two-thirds, and because of Miriam's age the baby is at higher risk of being a Down's baby and of being delivered prematurely. This is just the start of the potential problems.

A few pages back I was talking about my last OB call at the University last Saturday. One of the deliveries in which I participated that day was a woman in her mid-twenties who delivered twins at 24 weeks. The second baby was breech, which further complicated an already touch-and-go situation. While any baby delivered before 37 weeks is considered premature, those delivered after 32 weeks usually fare pretty well. When you go below 32, the morbidity and mortality statistics go way up, and given our current technology, the earliest gestational age at which we can sustain life outside the uterus is 24 weeks.

So these kids were at the edge. "Baby A" came out crying, which was, I thought, an unbelievably encouraging sign. Baby B fared less well, but both were still very much alive over a half hour later as the OB team was finishing up the work on mom, which included clearing the uterus of any retained placental products and sewing up a minor vaginal laceration. Mom and dad were smiling, crying tears of joy, hugging each other, grasping out to hold hands with nurses and other staff. It seemed like they couldn't be happier.

Maybe they really did understand how grave the situation was, but somehow their almost total show of happiness led me to think that they didn't completely fathom how bad a situation they were in. Because the chance that either of those kids will survive a month are about one in two, and the odds that they'll reach childhood "intact" — that is, without severe neurologic or physiologic impairments such as blindness, deafness, retardation and cerebral palsy — are about one in twenty.

I do not like those odds. I do not want to be in that situation.

Maybe I'm looking at this the wrong way, and that I should just take the plunge and have faith that things will work out. After all, it's not like the worrying is going to stop in the event that I have a "normal" child; the worry of having something wrong occur during pregnancy is going to be replaced by the worry for an infant's welfare, and later for a child's welfare, and eventually for a teen's welfare. The worrying will never stop. Still, I think I'd have just a little peace-of-mind if I knew that we will get through the next nine months okay.

On the subject of pregnant white women with decent incomes, good jobs, and generous health-care plans, I couldn't believe how different Santakis's office practice is from the women at the COC clinic. I knew it would be different — the COC patients are almost exclusively Medicaid, mostly black women, many unemployed and uneducated, adjectives that describe none of the women I saw today — but I was stunned at just *how* different. Even when I saw patients in private practice in Family Medicine, Pediatrics, and Internal Medicine, I was located in parts of town where much of those docs' practices were based off lower-income workers with decent health benefits. Many of the patients were doing okay financially but weren't exactly living The Soft Life.

Not so the women walking through the door in Blue Ash. Blue Ash is a suburb with a large Jewish population, tremendously wealthy and highly educated, not unlike Shaker Heights in Ohio, Newton in Massachusetts, or Farmington Hills in Michigan. Making it to Blue Ash isn't hitting quite the home-run that owning a house in the ultra-exclusive Indian Hill would constitute, but I'd call it a stand-up triple in the game of life. As I was driving on the highway looking for his office this morning, I took a few wrong turns and ended up in what appeared to be the Sycamore Township square. It was the perfect picture of relatively well-heeled noveau riche suburbia: Crisply manicured city-park lawns with not a hint of trash anywhere in sight; newly-paved sidewalks (but the abundant parking lots indicated that they were more for show than use); and buildings that were, by my reckoning, less than twenty years old, not yet showing their age, and simply awful to look at. As I managed to turn my car around, I thought, Toto, we're not in Kansas anymore.

The women coming to the medical office building about three blocks away from the town square were a product of this environment, and despite my contempt for suburbia I mean that in a complimentary way. Almost every one of the pregnant women that I saw today were having babies that they *planned* on having. They had the means to support these children, and had been taking care of their bodies so that the babies would be gestating in the most physiologically welcoming environment possible. They had been reading up on what they should expect from their obstetrician in various women's journals, the internet, and books that they snapped up at the local Barnes and Noble. In short, they were so distant from the women coming to the COC clinic that *that* practice might as well be in Senegal.

Still, America *is* America, and as utterly foreign as Blue Ash is from the slums of Cincinnati, similarities still creep in at the margins. Unfortunately, these similarities are of the less pleasant variety…

Santakis and I walked in to see a patient. I feel like I've gotten pretty good at instant vibe-readings from patients as the year has gone on, and I pretty much trust my gut when something seems amiss. In this case, what seemed amiss was that the mother, a salt-and-pepper-haired woman in her late 30s and maybe thirty- or forty-pounds overweight, was sitting on the exam table in the standard demeaning "paper gown" that I've seen used for women for breast and gyn exams. The top is like a cowboy vest made out of a thin plastic with a paper cover; the bottom is a wrap-around which covers one adequately in the front and not at all in the back. They look pretty humiliating to wear; I guess you could make a case that they're necessary to expedite the physical exam.*

Anyway, *that* wasn't the problem. The problem was that she was sitting there, ready for a full breast and pelvic exam, with her four year-old son sitting right there in the room. I wanted very much to escort the boy out of the room, but saw that it wasn't my call to make, that Santakis was acting as if there was no problem with his attendance. Maybe I'm wrong in thinking that he shouldn't have been there, but any doubt that she was a bit strange vanished over the next several minutes as I listened to her chat with Santakis about the goings-on in her life, which included her recent divorce from her husband, and how very glad she was to have him out of her life, since she passionately hated him. What she had to say didn't make me

---

* But would a *woman* be behind the invention of such a gown? I think not!

think her strange so much as that she was willing to carry on this discussion with the boy right there.

We came out of the exam room and made it back to the confines of his office. Santakis looked at me and winked. "She's a little cuckoo, no?" he said. "A sweet woman, but still a touch odd."

I nodded.

"Her husband tried to kill her, you know."

"You mean, *really* tried to kill her?"

"Oh yes. Very much."

I let a moment or two pass while he scribbled some notes. I thought about how often he got involved in domestic violence issues, and if he ever had to serve in a capacity above and beyond the strictly "medical" part of being a physician and call the cops. "Doctor Santakis," I said a few moments later. "Do you ever—"

"—I certainly *do*," was his immediate reply, clearly anticipating the question. "One time I had this lady from Indian Hill—Indian Hill!—and she comes in, and she's acting *really* strange. She isn't usually like this, and I'm thinking, 'what the hell's going on with her today?' So I start talking to her, and I get her a little calmed down, and I find out that she had just been in a fight with her husband before she came over to see me, and her husband put a gun to her head. He wanted to shoot her."

"Jesus!" was all I could say, feeling sharp about delivering such a zippy comeback. "What'd you do?"

"Called the police. I didn't have much of a choice," he replied. "You don't call the police in a situation like that, when someone's obviously in trouble, *you* could end up in a world of trouble."

Well, it's good to see that the inner-city has no corner on the market of misery.

Wednesday, June 13

I like Dr. Santakis a lot. I am going to try to see if Miriam would be interested in having Dr. Santakis deliver the baby, is how much I like him. I have fun when I'm in his office, and it's obvious that many of his patients like his easygoing but to-the-point style. He's got a very busy schedule, both in the obstetric and gynecologic end of his practice, so apparently there aren't too many women who are weirded out by the prospect of having a male gynecologist. All in all, it's been a pleasant two-week ride.

That said, I do *nothing*. I mean, literally, nothing. I follow him around as he sees the patients, sit and watch as he performs the exams, sit and listen as he talks to them. I do *not* perform any examinations myself — no paps, no pelvics, no fundal palpations on pregnant women. Because I like him so much, and because I have no interest in becoming a gynecologist, I don't make much of a fuss about it. Still, there's no question that this is not the optimal learning environment.

A good experience as a third-year requires lots of hands-on projects. It's easy to sit and watch people do their work, but you don't really learn anything as you go, because once you try to do the tasks that they perform with ease — whether it's thinking about what drugs to give someone or throwing knots in a surgery — you realize that it ain't so easy. I'm aware that I'm not revealing anything earthshaking, but it underscores how difficult it can be when, as a third-year, you encounter a preceptor that doesn't give you room to learn. Had I not liked Santakis, or had I any desire to be an obstetrician, I'd be going absolutely straight out of my gourd.

Saturday, June 16   on-call

My final part of the OB/GYN rotation is doing gynecologic surgery at the Christ Hospital. It's nice to have come full circle and finish the year where I started it. I came up on to the 10th floor to the call rooms on my first day back and saw all of the dead Miller-moths and entered my forty-five degree call room and thought, "yeah, it's good to be back."

The gynecologic surgery suites on the 8th floor of Christ look very much like the general surgery ORs down in the bowels of the building. The ORs are in use by many different private-practice docs, and thus there's constant turnover from about 7:30 a.m. until about 2 p.m., when things tend to peter out a bit.

That said, the difference between the gyn surgeons and general surgeons working ten floors below couldn't be more pronounced. With one or two exceptions, everyone that I've worked with is pleasant—and not just to residents, but to the entire team. One surgeon came in one day and saw a scrub tech that he hadn't worked with before. "Hi, I'm Rick," said the doctor as he held out his hand. It was the first time all year that I ever heard a physician introduce himself or herself without the title "doctor" in front of it.

Not only are the surgeons more pleasant, but the entire tone of the OR is more mellow, less anxiety-provoking. A lot of this I think is due to the overwhelming female presence. *All* of the residents are women. Plus some of the attendings are women as well. Yesterday I was doing a hysterectomy with Dr. Sarnak, a mid-forties gyn oncologist, and Denise Samson, a third-year resident. The chit-chat through the first hour of surgery was about their children, who were seven years and twenty months old, respectively. The second hour focused intensely on Denise's haircut, and whether or not her hairdresser committed malpractice by not tailoring her hair to look like Jamie Lee Curtis's. (For what it's worth, I thought the haircut did indeed look like the picture of JLC that Denise was showing everyone days before.) I thought to myself, well, there's the difference between your general surgeons and your gynecologists: The surgeons talk about their stereos and cars, the gynecologists talk about their kids and their haircuts. The haircut conversation rather put me to sleep, but still I'd hang with the gynecologists any day over the general surgeons for the quality of the shop-talk.

Being back at Christ is also eye-opening in terms of my understanding of how hospitals work. When I came here, all hospitals seemed alike to me: After all, how can one *really* evaluate which hospitals are better than others in terms of general patient care? Of course, there are specific reasons why one would want to be at one hospital over another. If you need a liver transplant, you're not going anywhere other than the U, and if you have a high-risk pregnancy and your babies may need a mega-high-tech nursery with the ability to care for a preemie, you need to be at the U or at Good Sam, and not at Jewish or Mercy Fairfield. But if you are coming in for bread-and-butter medicine (a coronary artery bypass, a routine delivery), it shouldn't matter in theory where you go. The nurses and doctors should be, on average, every bit as competent and caring as their colleagues at different hospitals.

I still believe that's mostly true, but I'm beginning to see subtle gradations that can change one's experience in a hospital. I asked Santakis what facility he recommended for delivering our baby. "They've all got advantages and disadvantages," he said. "You want the best nursery, then Good Sam is probably the best place to go." (Dr. Santakis did not include the University, although the U has an equally impressive nursery, because he has generally had bad experiences in his relationships with the hospital as a private practicioner. This is true of many private-practice doctors.) "You want the nicest rooms, then Mercy's great. You want anesthesia there in an instant, come here to Christ. I mean, when you're at the University, you'll ask for anesthesia to come and give an epidural, and you could wait until next week. You ask for an epidural at Christ, and the anesthesiologist will be on the phone with you instantly saying, 'I'll have it in forty seconds, and I'll be there in five minutes.'"

Miriam will be delivering baby Hatch-Tuchman at The Christ Hospital, largely but not entirely on the importance of the observation about anesthesia.

Tuesday, June 19

For me, gyn surgery consists largely of standing around the operating table doing nothing at all, even though I'm fully gowned and gloved, theoretically able to assist. At least in general surgery I either drove the laparoscopic camera or I retracted, and usually I assisted in closing. In gyn surgery, I do nothing at all. Nobody pimps me, nobody asks me to do anything. How on earth we're supposed to be evaluated I have no idea, but essentially I don't care. I mean, I'm not looking to make any trouble, but if they aren't aggressive about educating me, it's not like I'm going into surgery, so why bother?

Every once in a while, though, they surprise me. One young doc casually asked me, in the middle of an abdominal hysterectomy, if I knew the venous drainage of the left ovary, and without even thinking about it I answered the left renal vein, which was absolutely right. *How* I managed to call up that little bit of obscure information, two and a half years away from my anatomy class, is completely beyond me. Everyone in the room seemed pleased with my answer; I nearly fainted from having pulled it out so nonchalantly.

And then there are moments when I realize that, although in two weeks I will be taking that quantum leap into the fourth year by starting my acting internship, I'm still that retarded, awkward third-year whom everyone gets to rib. I had been called out of one surgery that I was observing so that I could observe an ovarian tumor removal performed by Dr. Walsh in another suite. Walsh wanted any available student who wasn't scrubbed in to come take a look, and I was the only student who wasn't sterile. I soon realized why she asked for us: This was a tumor, in a little old lady, the size of a *football.*

Then she asked me to grab a bucket so that she could remove the tumor and we could send it to pathology. I turned around and found a plastic bucket, and brought it to the level of the operating table. "No, I can't have it that close, we'll lose the sterile field," she said. So I placed the bucket on the floor and she said, "No, just bring it up halfway." I was holding the bucket on each side, which had no handles, by my thumb and forefinger, and as she dropped the tumor from two feet above, I realized much too late that I wouldn't be able to keep my grasp on the bucket as the roughly ten-pound weight hit it.

The bucket shot straight to the floor, and out bounced the tumor, dribbling underneath the operating table. Everyone was silent, but it didn't take a genius to realize that absolutely everyone in that room was trying with all their collective might to keep from laughing hysterically. Naturally, I felt stupid, and got on my knees to crawl under the table to pick it up.

"Hey, don't worry about getting it," one of the OR techs said. "I'll just kick it on down to pathology."

Wednesday, June 20

Tomorrow I have my oral examination, and Friday I have the written exam, and then my third year is officially over, coming in precisely the way I left, with an oral and a written. I can tell you this: I am substantially less prepared for these examinations than I was for the general surgery exams, or any other exam this year (with the possible exception of Family Medicine). Only providence will allow me to sail through and emerge without tanking my final grade in OB/GYN.

I could blame this lack of preparation on a host of factors: The excitement of gearing up for the Acting Internship; the excitement of learning that my wife is pregnant; the added excitement of learning that there are *twins* hanging out in there.

But the real reason is much more mundane: Pure apathy. I've just become too tired of showing up and playing Mister Happy-To-Be-Here when, in fact, I'm ready to begin focusing on my future specialty of internal medicine. Do I *really* want to memorize the cardinal movements of labor? Not particularly. Do I need to have a thorough understanding of the anatomy of the female reproductive system? No thanks. Just tell me the parts I need for a career in Medicine and I'll move on.

This is not a good attitude to have if you want to curry favor with the residents and attendings, as I've said before. But it's even more poisonous as exam time nears, especially as the summer begins, because it's difficult enough to sit down and study for long hours after a full day's work; it's that much more difficult when you're not especially motivated. And this is why I will not get honors in OB/GYN unless the course director happens to be sucking nitrous oxide when he fills in the gradesheet.

Thursday, June 21

"Hi, Doctor Schwarz," I say earlier this morning as I offer my hand in introduction, opening his office door. "I'm your next student for the oral exam."

"Oh, hi there," he says.

"Hey—is that a *Brandeis* banner?"

"It sure is. I went there for undergraduate. Why do you ask?"

"I did, too."

"Really?"

"Yeah. When'd you graduate?"

"Nineteen eighty-nine."

This guy is two years older than me. I regard this as a serious bummer, but I have every intention of using it to my advantage, which I need since I'm deeply unprepared for what's to come.

"Cool. I haven't run into anyone from the alma mater since I've moved here," I say.

"Yeah, that is neat."

"Listen, before we start, can I ask you a question?"

"Sure."

"How long does this take? Since we're running a bit behind, I was just wondering, because I've got a doctor's appointment." He was actually running an *hour* behind examining other students, but I was all peaches & cream in my tone.

"Oh? Is everything okay?"

"Yeah, it's fine actually. I have to go to an OB appointment with my wife. We just found out she's pregnant with twins."

"Really!"

Time to use this to my advantage. "Yeah, it's been really hard to concentrate over the last couple of days. I'm afraid I'm going to make a mess of this test."

"That's great news. Would you rather take it next week sometime?"

With the end of my third year slated for *tomorrow*? Not a chance, baby. "Oh, no, that's okay, I don't think I'm going to be any better off in a few days. I'll just take it as it comes today and deal with it."

"Well, we'll try to get you out of here quickly enough so that you can go be with your wife, and we'll make it as painless as possible."

Gotcha.

Not that what I was saying wasn't true, but I figured I needed to pull out the stops just in case I had a shot at Honors. I'm reasonably certain I don't, but I also don't want to end up with a *pass*, which in this class amounts to near-failure, so inflated is the grading system.

The exam wasn't that bad at all, and based on what I heard from classmates in the hallway it wasn't substantially different from their own orals. He gave me three clinical situations and asked me how to work the patient up. One was ovarian cancer, another was breast cancer — both conditions that I knew how to work up. The third question was about managing the workup of a young woman with hormonal dysfunction, and unfortunately I didn't stick the landing. Still, I don't think I tanked it, and I was very worried about doing just that earlier this morning, when I awoke in a cold sweat, aware that I was seriously underprepared for the exam.

Tomorrow I will take the written exam, but I can already tell you how it's going to go. I'll get questions about the cardinal movements, about the various forms of contraception and their efficacy rates, about uterine leiomyomas, about Asherman's Syndrome, and about various other goodies that affect the female reproductive system. I will probably get about four out of five questions right, and that, in conjunction with my oral and my decidedly average clinical performance on this clerkship, will equal a high-pass. I'm going to finish almost exactly the way I came in when I took Step One: On a nice, easy coast. But in between those two unimpressive markers in my career, I had my pedal on the floor, and I'm proud of that.

And that, as they say, is all, folks.

epilogue:

April 2002

For those who are pondering medical school:

So, you still wanna go through with this?

Well, bully for you, I say. I don't have any regrets about this career choice, and I've tasted different flavors of jobs before I got here—teaching English, washing dishes, writing science articles, yes, even raising turkeys. I don't yet know whether or not I will like being a doctor, but I've loved medical school, and whatever unpleasant things I may have experienced and written about don't diminish my belief that this is a great profession, a noble calling, and an intellectual adventure.

So, by all means, go for it. Just know what you're getting yourself into. My experience was not fundamentally different from that of most third-years in medical schools across the United States. No matter where you are, you still experience the same sense of unavoidable humiliation, some of it earned, some of it not; you still feel the same terror when you see your first patient crash; you still sweat the exams; and you still can smell the air of competition between your classmates, no matter how much you all like one another and try to help each other survive. If what I wrote makes you think that you don't want to live through that, think about law school instead. Keep in mind, though, that their hours often suck just as much, and they're usually doing things far less interesting than what we get to do. And we *help* people at the end of the day.

To do medical school well, or at least to do the third year well, requires religious adherence to about five key rules, and in my opinion you're sunk without them. Roughly they go like this, in descending order of importance:

1. *Laugh at yourself.* Laugh a lot, because in your third year you are a bumbling, fucking idiot. I'm only finishing my fourth year; soon I'll be a "real" doctor—and I'll be only slightly less dumb. Get used to giving the wrong answer in front of ten people who know more than you. And not just wrong answers, but *whacked* answers. Prepare yourself for stuttering, stammering, fumbling your way through presentations, day after day, often with less sympathetic people quietly chuckling at your stellar ignorance. They *should* be laughing because it *is* funny—and it's a pretty magical transformation from being a

third-year goofball to becoming the machine of efficiency and confidence that a resident becomes by, say, the beginning of his or her second or third year.

Above all else, the only quality that will sustain you through that period of professional nascence, when nearly everything you do is embarrassingly wrong, is the ability to laugh at yourself.

2. *Give a damn.* To my mind, this is the most important piece of being a good doctor overall, but it ranks second during the third year. Giving a damn about your patients and their lives has dramatic implications for your success as a med student. It will help you study better if you know what you have to learn to take care of them (and that's usually a staggering amount) and it will make that information easier to remember if you can associate it with a patient.

Moreover, good docs recognize and reward students who care. Most everyone will understand if you're eager to cut loose on a Friday afternoon if they see you take a genuine interest in what's happening on Friday *morning*, or if they see that you will follow-up with a patient even after you leave your rotation. Sometimes, because you move through the system so rapidly, you are in fact *better* situated to help patients once you're finished with a rotation than the very docs who teach you.

For instance, when I did my pediatrics rotation in February, I encountered a patient that clearly needed a child psychiatrist, but needed to work with someone who didn't charge much. Dr. Blumstein was hard pressed to think of a kid shrink that would operate on the sliding scale that this family needed, but I placed a call to "Doctor Bob" Tomlinson's office and tried to find out if he could see this girl through the residents' child psych clinic. The plan worked, and as of the last time I talked to Blumstein they had made the arrangements for her to be evaluated at Children's Hospital. That may have been the single most important thing I did last year, because only I had that knowledge of the system and its players simply because I was getting to see the medical panorama and wasn't locked into my own specialty and my own contacts.

3. *Hustle.* Hustle like your ass is on fire. Do what you say you're going to do. The adage for the surgery clerkship is, "Be at the hospital before the residents arrive and leave after the last resident is walking out the door," and while that's a *bit* overkill, it expresses the sentiment quite nicely. Your world-class sense of humor aside, the most important thing to sustain the grind, especially the sense that what you're doing is just following people around a lot and pretending to act like you know what you're doing when you don't have a clue, is to approach each day with the kind of energy you put into your fantasy league, or your wedding, or your church outing, whatever revs your engine.

Based on my own impressions, the students who don't perform as well during third year are the ones who decide to take lunch before checking up on a patient's labs before reporting back to the resident, or the ones who ask, "Now when exactly can I go home?" One of those students was a good friend of mine, and I saw her run into the same problem with residents on virtually every one of her clerkships. When it first happened, during Surgery, I chalked it up to those silly surgeons, but when it happened again, and again, and eleven months later I heard OB/GYN residents voicing the *same* complaints about her preoccupation with not being around, I couldn't help but conclude there was a trend. (More on patterns anon.)

4. *Know your job.* It took me well over six months to realize that a third-year's job is simple: You need to learn how to take a patient's history, perform an adequate physical exam, present the patient's case to the medical team, and exhibit the qualities mentioned above. It's much less important to "do procedures" such as inserting a central line, or help close during a surgery, or be the one to help prep a patient before they get cut. It's nice if you get to do those things, but that shouldn't be the main goal. You may run to radiology faster than anyone else on the team, and you can offer to help stick an NG tube down a patient as many times as you want, but if you don't prepare and practice your presentations the night before Your Big Moment and then you stumble, you won't get a good grade and you don't

deserve it. Stick to the basics: History, physical, presentation. Nobody expects you to know a lot. Indeed, nobody expects you to know *anything*, because, and I hope I haven't belabored this point, you don't.

The single biggest mistake I made during my third year was not keeping this in mind, or even not understanding this until late in the game. I spent a lot of time looking up articles to present to attendings, thinking this was going to look so impressive, when I should have been up practicing my presentation and reading about the basics of my patients' conditions. I ended up looking silly — like somehow *I'm* gonna provide someone with ten, fifteen more years training than me a totally new way of looking at things because of one little article from the New England Journal of Medicine — and it smacked of the kind of sycophantic behavior I was originally determined to avoid.

I can state with a fair amount of confidence that what prevented me from getting Honors in Pediatrics was *one* poor presentation at the beginning of my inpatient month. All of my other evaluations were excellent, and I did reasonably well on the test. The difference between earning distinction and staying with the pack amounted to five bungled minutes out of two months. Had I decided on pediatrics for my residency, that would have been a very big deal, indeed, for it would have all but closed off any chance I might have had at the more competitive programs. *Five minutes.* And because of it, I didn't receive Honors. And I didn't deserve it.

5. *Never, ever complain in front of anyone, other than classmates.* You're not a victim. You shouldn't complain at all, because being a third-year medical student on the way to a very financially sound career doesn't give you much room to bitch. But let's be serious, and honor Joe Walsh's dictum: I can't complain, but sometimes I still do. Living through the third year means even the hospital *janitor* can boss you and your 3.7 college-educated butt around — so it's natural to whine a little or a lot as the punches roll your way. I wasn't immune, for it's not very hard to find evidence of it in the preceding pages.

However — don't *ever* do it in front of a resident, fellow, or attending! They don't want to hear about your tough life! They don't want to hear about people that you don't like! During my OB/GYN clerkship, in the middle of the night on Labor & Delivery, when it was quiet, the residents and students were hanging around in the lounge munching on takeout. Since we students were deciding on which residencies we were going to pursue, the residents were asking us about our choices.

"What do you think?" one of the residents asked me.

"I think I'm a medicine guy," I said plainly.

"Don't like obstetrics and gynecology?" he returned.

"No, it's not that. I like it *all*," I replied truthfully. "I'd do all of them if I could."

"Not so much for the surgical end of things? Is that it?"

"Exactly. It's cool stuff, but not for me. I mean, I *loved* surgery, but I'm more…"

"Oh my *God*," my classmate Dara interrupted. "I *hated* surgery. It *sucked!*"

The resident raised his eyebrows and put his finger to his lips, like musing over what his next move in the chess game would be. "Why, exactly, did it suck?" he asked.

"Because they're a bunch of *tyrants!*" Dara responded. "I mean, I was watching a surgery once, and the attending had to leave the room for a few minutes, and we were told to wait and not to close on the patient until he returned, even though the surgery was basically over. We waited and waited, and finally the resident said that's it, let's close him up. About halfway through the attending walked in and started screaming at us. I told him that we decided it was time to close him up when I saw the mold growing on the wound."

"So, um, you don't like them very much, do you?" the resident asked.

"Oh my God, surgeons just *suck!*" she said. "They're all a bunch of psychos!"

Does she realize that she's talking to a surgeon? I thought to myself. Does she realize that what the resident is almost certainly thinking is: What's she gonna say about *us* when she moves onto her next rotation? Bottom line: Keep your tongue in check unless you're around someone you know and trust.

Those are your basic rules. There are other minor ones:

Respect the hierarchy; always assist your classmates; take your lumps even when you're right and your critic is wrong. This last rule, I've discovered, can be tough for people who've been used to being "A" students their entire lives, and have been told repeatedly how superior they are to the rest of humanity. Take that kind of person and throw them into a group, and judge them directly against other students? Oh, there's bound to be trouble.

The simple principle that many third-years don't appreciate is the more you complain, the bigger you dig your hole. You increase the chance that there's somebody in the medical center who's going to be reluctant to do you a favor someday, and that mild criticism on an evaluation is not likely to be remembered by an attending at all, but one who *complains* about the injustice of that evaluation is much more likely to be remembered, permanently, as a bad apple.

I also realized halfway through the year that grades are a good deal more objective than most people realize. One of the major complaints of students (those not getting Honors) is that subjective grading is an unjust system, one entirely subject to the whim of whichever resident or attending is evaluating them, and one in which a student can take the hit because so-and-so is having problems at home, or isn't getting enough sleep, etc. Lunchtime griping about *this* grade or *that* evaluation was endemic.

After my surgery grades came back, I partially had this sensibility. I believed my evaluation from Scott the resident didn't reflect at all my assessment of my talents. Still, I thought, if Dr. Mittleschmertz says the same thing in Family Medicine, and then I see it again in psych, well then, there must be a *pattern* going on here. If you see one person knock you for something, it might just be a personality conflict. But if *all* of your evaluations are coming back in the "pass" range, isn't it more likely that you simply aren't an exceptional student?

By the middle of February, I knew I had my answer: Of all my clinical evaluations, which at that point numbered twelve, only *one* did not give me an honors-level grade. Only one failed to address my drive, my compassion, my brilliance, my Mother Theresa-like qualities. Overstatement? Sure. But no accident. I got too many good grades from too many different kinds of docs to chalk it up to luck.

ΩΩΩΩΩΩΩΩΩ

If you *aren't* planning on being a doc, and you're reading this:

I don't mean for this to be an exposé or to embarrass anyone at the medical school. I believe in what we're doing, and I mean for this to be an advertisement about what's mostly *good* in the medical system. The University of Cincinnati is a great medical center. Are there problems with our medical school, and does our profession need to take big strides at relating better to our patients? Absolutely. But that doesn't mean that there's any system that takes care of people's ailments better than what is foolishly called "Western medicine." Everything else, call it what you want, is quackery.

More than anything else, my third year of school has reinforced my belief that the options offered by science-based modern medicine are almost always the only real options that people have. Ranting aside, though, it's *true* that so many of the patients I wrote about aren't going to improve in terms of their health, and all of that fascinating Western science isn't going to do a whit to stop the degenerative processes destroying their bodies. The best we can do is engage in a holding action and stave off the inevitable, which often involves marked physical limitation or tremendous pain.

It's also true that many other patients I wrote about are victims of a social system rather than a particular medical ailment — and what we can offer is, at best, a band-aid for their afflictions. Bernie, the Child-Psych kid who ran a pencil through the hand of another child? *Five days* in the psych ward to "cure" a mildly retarded kid who's lived around violence all of his ten years? I don't think so. That's your future headline-grabbing gruesome-homicide perpetrator. The 16 year-old women (girls!) coming through OB with their third baby, who have no education, little family support, no father, and no income? Those are future social services case-files. The three-pack-a-day smoking, six-pack-a-day drinking vets whose toes and legs are getting amputated? There's your tax dollars at work, going to the deeply underfunded, understaffed VA nursing homes, for which there is a long waiting list.

For these people, the ones seen at public, city hospitals across the United States, much of what we medical students and residents do is simply bear witness to their misery. Whatever "medical" help we provide only touches on what really afflicts them. For many patients, the ones who *don't* have nice white-collar jobs in plush office parks with decent salaries and health-care benefits, the answers lie in the way our entire social structure is built, and they'll only have a chance if we dream of changing that structure from the foundation up.

Another impression that I certainly hope I didn't convey is that academic medical centers are more dangerous places than the luxurious private hospitals of the suburbs, where inexperienced interns and residents run amok with no supervision. I'm rather irritated by the articles I've noticed popping up in the past year or two written by interns or residents that show up in *Salon* or *The New Yorker* explaining how young doctor so-and-so has simply *no idea whatsoever* what he or she is doing. Moreover, people learn to their absolute *shock*, and nearly complete *horror*, that when under the knife, quietly resting with their guts literally exposed, there is a mere *resident* who's actually *practicing* on them!

Shut up, shut up. Hey people, guess what? *We need practice.* And guess what else? *It's not going to kill you.* When Joe Intern is in the OR, and an exquisitely trained surgeon is watching over his shoulder while he dissects away someone's grandpa's nerve so as not to molest it during his hernia repair, you better believe that they're getting the best care possible. Remember, Doctor Surgeon is standing right there, actually *running* the surgery, handling anything that's too complicated for the apprentice. I think sometimes people get the idea that the attending surgeon just checks out, saying, "Hey guys, I'll be at the golf course! Call if there's any trouble!" and waddles out of the room. This isn't how it works, for the quality control in surgery is very, very tight.

In medical (i.e. nonsurgical) fields the situation of resident supervision is a bit different, but the impact of being in an academic medical center on patient's health is perhaps even more profound. You go to some suburban private hospital for your chest pain, Doctor Private-Practice will see you at six in the morning for maybe five minutes while en route to work. *Maybe* if you're lucky he or she will see you when going home as well. That's a max of ten minutes per day. If there's anything tricky about your management, Doctor Private-Practice has to take care of it by phone, talking to the nurse from his or her office halfway across town. He or she can't see you, can't talk to you, can't *examine* you. If that nurse isn't vigilant, you could be in a world of hurt.

Now, if you're that same patient at an academic medical center, here's what you might encounter: A medical student will see you, talk to you, and examine you. Then an intern, who got the report from the student, will also visit you so as to determine for themselves the nature of your ailment. *Then* the senior resident will drop by to check you out. Finally, the formal rounds will be made with the attending and any ideas as to what's going on are going to be kicked around. You've gotten, for the same price as the private hospital, *four* different people thinking about your problem and discussing it with each other. Moreover, at least two of those four people (the student and intern) will be in your room two, three, even four times everyday just checking in to see how you're doing. You are watched over *very* carefully when a resident takes care of you. So take a deep breath and don't worry. You're going to do just fine with the residents. (Most of them, anyway.)

ΩΩΩΩΩΩΩΩΩ

If I could sum up what I learned during my third year in only two sentences, this is how it would look.

Sentence #1: Smoking is bad for you. You knew that already, now didn't you? But not like I know it. People can eat poorly and ruin their hearts; they can drink and wreak havoc on their livers; and they can sit around and watch TV all day and fatten themselves right into diabetes. They can smoke crack, and they can have unprotected sex with lots of partners. But, from a public-health perspective, none of these practices have the kind of impact that smoking cigarettes does. I saw more cases of people with emphysema and chronic bronchitis than I care to remember during the past two years, and I'm going to see lots more of it in internal medicine. Get fifty percent of smokers to stop and those two conditions would become a lot less common.

Watching smokers decline is a terrible thing to behold. As they lose their lung tissue, they become increasingly dependent on technology that enables them to breathe. At first, they can be helped with medications alone like, say, ipratroprium, but eventually, they become dependent on oxygen canisters that they cart around with them. Finally, they start to bounce in and out of the hospital as they become occasionally dependent on ventilators.

I've come to realize that what most doctors really do is help a patient preserve his or her *quality* of life rather than simply save the patient's life itself. Big-time smokers that come to rely on doctors and their medicines, by my reckoning, have the crappiest quality of life when compared to other patients with nasty chronic disorders, such as heart-bypass or kidney-dialysis patients who don't smoke. And doctors can't do a whole lot to improve their lot in life, except give more oxygen.

There's a lot of suffering out there that doctors are currently powerless to stop. We can't do a whole lot for people with rheumatoid arthritis or lupus. But I find it almost criminal that people willingly subject themselves to poison on a daily basis over decades of time only to become *deliberately reliant* on doctors and medicines. It is a totally preventable, and absolutely unnecessary practice. If I learned a lesson last year it was that tobacco companies should be every physician's sworn enemy.

I won't even begin to tell you how I feel when I see a select number of my classmates smoke. They should be thrown out of school.

Sentence #2: The single most important factor in the education of US medical students and residents are the Veterans of the Armed

Forces of the United States. You cannot measure the contribution that vets make, so important is their donation. This isn't a phenomenon restricted to southern Ohio. I don't know the precise figures, but a large number of medical schools across the US have affiliations with their local VAs, which in turn rely on the students and residents. Theoretically everyone wins: Apprentice docs have greater responsibilities than elsewhere; the VA gets for essentially free a large labor pool in students and residents; vets that might not otherwise have health insurance receive quality care.

When I was looking at residency programs last fall, I went to New Hampshire to interview at the Dartmouth-Hitchcock Medical Center. Like many University-based programs, Dartmouth has a VA component to its medical education. When one of the chief residents was giving a slide show extolling the virtues of his program, he stopped when the picture of the VA hospital came up and asked us if we came from medical schools that had affiliations with VAs. About three-quarters of us raised our hands.

"Yeah, I figured that," he said. "Well, then I'm sure it won't come as a surprise to you when I say that you absolutely *must* get some training, either as a medical student or resident, at a program that has a VA experience."

Truer words have never been spoken.

ΩΩΩΩΩΩΩΩΩ

The change between the third year and fourth year is almost as dramatic as the one between second and third year. People treat you differently — partly because everyone knows that your main focus is on doing the residency dance. That means you are either taking a course that will help you get into the residency of your choice (known to fourth-years as "How hard can I work in one month?") or you are taking what is officially known as an "elective" (known to fourth-years as "Um, when can I leave?").

At UC, the fourth-years are required to take two months of Acting Internship in Internal Medicine. Since I had decided on that fateful day just about a year ago to go into Internal Medicine, the AIs were critical clerkships, and consequently I top-loaded my schedule in the fourth year: Two AIs and a month of Infectious Disease. Those would be the last grades to show up on my residency application transcript, and it was absolutely essential that I didn't make a mess of things or I could kiss going to Boston or the competitive northeast goodbye. I *had* to get Honors on at least one of those AIs.

My first AI was at the University Hospital, and by the end I knew that *this* month would have been the perfect subject for a book. What a month it was. Every image you can conjure up about a bad medical experience — an arrogant and boorish attending physician, an intern so frightfully incompetent that it was a miracle nobody was killed under his service, a pair of oft-terrified wide-eyed third-years, a ward floor whose nursing was so ridiculously bad that all the residents routinely referred to it as the "Death Star" — I lived it for 33 days in June and July. Had it not been for my fellow AI and team leader, both of whom managed to keep me laughing during what was almost daily hell with the attending, I almost certainly would have committed some unspeakable act.

Somehow, astonishingly, against all odds, and likely the result of some heavy-duty lobbying on the part of my team leader, I walked away with Honors for the rotation. I was certain that the attending physician didn't like me or my hyper-kinetic style, and didn't think much of my abilities. I dreaded the meeting when he gave me my evaluation, quietly whispering to myself as I walked toward his office to *stay calm, don't object and just get out of there*...but then the moment arrived and he turned into this different beast, all smiles and congratulations, telling me that this-and-that aspect of my game was, of all things, excellent. I offered my thanks to him and the team leader, and wandered out of the office, utterly stunned by what had happened.

By contrast, my second AI, at the Christ Hospital, was almost criminally easy. At the University, I slept, if I was lucky, three hours when I was on call. At Christ, I *walked home* if I was finished with my patients by 10 p.m. on call nights! My

Christ team leader was impressed when I would go and check peripheral blood smears on my patients without being told to do so; if I didn't do that at the University, someone would kick my ass halfway to the moon. I received Honors for the Christ AI in what felt like a runaway. I enjoyed the month so much that I even briefly flirted with the idea of departing from my University-bound career and instead doing my residency at Christ. Briefly, anyway. But in my heart, I knew I was University-bound. A community-based program wouldn't do.

During these early pseudo-intern experiences I've learned to appreciate the critical role that nurses play in patient care, and the wide differences in nursing talent across the medical specialties. The Death Star was the second most terrifying thing I observed throughout medical school (second only to that bungling intern). I repeatedly had to check on orders that I had written to make sure they were carried out; often medications weren't administered, but could be found just lying around the central supply area, there for the taking. Once I had a very sick patient there who had a morning potassium level of 2.5, which is dangerously low, and basically constitutes an emergency. I immediately wrote an order for a large dose of potassium to be administered through a central line and called my senior to have him verify the order to the nurse (since fourth-years, who aren't licensed, cannot give orders without a resident's approval). This needed to be taken care of within the hour. After making sure that the nurse took the order and knew to look for the potassium coming from the pharmacy, I headed off to the other side of the hospital to take care of my other patients. I returned two hours later to the patient's room and there's *no potassium*. I practically dashed to the central storage, and there it was, lying on the counter. When I found the nurse, I was furious.

"Well, I was busy doing other things," she said without much concern.

That patient could easily have died. I call that bad nursing.

At the other extreme, I developed a tremendous respect for Intensive Care Unit nurses. They are the Marines of the nursing corps: The most dedicated, the most competent, the ones who you can count on to get things done because things *have* to be done. While an AI, several of my patients ended up getting "bounced" into the ICU, and though the ICU team would take care of them, the ward team would follow along, in preparation for taking them once they bounced out of the ICU and into a halfway house known as the Step-Down unit on their way back to the wards. Both the ICU and Step-Down nurses were scary in their no-bullshit efficiency and their medical knowledge, which often rivaled the interns and residents, so thorough their training had been. I never had a concern about one of my orders being followed in the Step-Down.

ΩΩΩΩΩΩΩΩΩ

I can't do justice to the residency dance in a few paragraphs. It really deserves its own chapter, but I didn't have the heart to write anything after third year: That was my end point, and when I reached it I didn't even look at a keyboard for six months. During that time I was practicing my pirouettes and pliés for interview season. I followed the interview trail to thirteen programs: By my reckoning, two of the programs were extremely competitive, nine were competitive academic programs, and two were private hospitals I regarded as safety programs in case I tanked. About ten other programs offered me interviews, but I turned them down, feeling confident about my chances. Another half-dozen or so didn't offer me interviews, including the Harvard hospitals, which my superiors had prophesied would likely happen.

Incidentally, submitting nearly thirty program applications — as a candidate in internal medicine — is considered ludicrous. I quote that much-read tome, *First Aid for the Match*, on applying to medicine residencies: "There are no hard and fast rules about the number of applications you should complete; however, some residency advisors suggest that the typical student send in 10 to 15 applications in order to secure interviews at 8 to 10 programs." I wasn't taking any chances after what my "advisors" told me about my competitiveness, but the more dire predictions turned out not to be accurate, and I had plenty of solid university programs to look at.

This is just a guess, but I think that medical students put much more stock in the interviews than do programs. When I was interviewing at a major academic program in Chicago, I decided to get bold with one of my interviewers, and asked him *exactly* how they figured out their rank list.

"You mean, no one's told you?"

"No, not really."

"Oh, it never occurred to me that you wouldn't know that. It's not a secret or anything. You know that an interview can only hurt you, right?"

"Uh, not exactly."

"And that letters of recommendation can only hurt you, right?"

"This is all news to me." The other applicants agreed.

"Well, here's what we do: After we've gone through the whole interview season, there's a big, long meeting on a Saturday in early February. We start at like eight in the morning and go pretty late into the night. There's lots of Chinese food, let me tell you. Anyway, we start out with a computer-generated list, with everyone ranked one to whatever, and beside them is a numeric value. We calculate that value by assigning points to various categories. You earn so many points for Honors in medicine, so many for a high-pass and pass. You earn points for your class rank and your board scores. We then assign an overall value to the reputation of your medical school — you know, students from Duke get a higher value than those from some state school — and multiply the points by the reputation factor. Once that overall value is assigned we have a tentative list. Then we look through the list and drop anybody who behaved badly during the interview day or had tepid letters of recommendation.

"But those things don't really *help* you. We assume that your letter writers are going to say that you're the next Albert Schweitzer and are capable of walking on water, and we take for granted that you know how to conduct yourself professionally and are able to interact appropriately with other human beings. The people who don't interview well go to the bottom of the list. Anyway, we take the remaining names, and everyone will lobby for someone they really like a lot to move up the list. That's what takes the longest time during the ranking session. Mostly, though, your spot on the list is already predetermined."

"Oh." I wondered what number they assigned for the reputation value of the University of Cincinnati.

What constitutes poor behavior on the part of a candidate? The following story comes from a classmate who matched in a surgical subspecialty on the east coast. At the interview, the candidates were sitting in a conference room, awaiting their interviewers. While there, one of the faculty, an American of Korean descent, dropped by and decided to introduce himself and tell them a little about his background. He mentioned that, in his youth, he fought in the Vietnam war.

"For which side?" said one of the candidates jokingly.

The doctor turned pale, looked around, and quickly left the room. The candidate, who was beginning to realize that his joke wasn't entirely appropriate based on the incredulous stares coming from the other applicants, said, "It's a *joke*, you see—I was joking." He was greeted with more stares, and, understanding that he had totally trampled the polite social atmosphere of the morning, stood up, gathered his belongings and hastily left. This was the smartest action to take, for there wasn't any point in his staying. He certainly wasn't going to make it onto that program's rank list.

Interviewing was much more tiring than I had expected it to be. This was due in part to the fact that I had not taken any "vacation" time to interview, but instead kept taking fourth-year electives (including a month at the Intensive Care Unit, where I went directly from a call night to New York City to look at a few programs in Manhattan). After the first few programs, the excitement wore off, and it became a grind.

That said, each time I looked at a new place—especially when I was in a new city—I got to imagine a different life for myself. If I matched at Dartmouth-Hitchcock, the snow-covered hills of New Hampshire would offer a much different life than the asphalt jungle of New York City if I matched at one of the Manhattan programs. All kinds of different cities were in the mix: Chicago, Providence, Cleveland, Philly, Columbus, not to mention the idea of staying on my home turf of Cincinnati. *That's* the exciting part of the match game: You really can go almost wherever you choose.

Where did I end up? Well, let's just say that the prophecies about Harvard were right, but I *was* a competitive candidate in the supposedly go-go northeast and I'm going to be at a University-based academic program in Boston, which was the plan all along. I'm happy with my choice. In fact, I would have been happy with any of my top nine choices. *That's* having good options.

All in all, it was a good run. I owed much of my good fortune to my decent showing during third year. Next stop, internship.

ΩΩΩΩΩΩΩΩΩ

Andrea, my classmate who was with me for all my courses during third year, matched into a community-based program in ER. Her advisors in the ER program had advised her to apply to at least thirty programs as they were concerned about her competitiveness in ER's increasingly popular applicant pool, where even community programs can snag good students. As with me, this proved to be an overkill piece of advice: She interviewed at an ungodly number of programs, nearly twenty in all, and got her first choice.

Vikash didn't make his mind up about what specialty he wanted to pursue, so he ended up applying to programs in urology, general surgery, and medicine. He decided to participate in the "early match" for urology that takes place in January (a few minor specialties don't participate in the "main" Match for various reasons). Vikash interviewed at a half-dozen urology programs on the east coast, and matched. This in theory should have resolved his dilemma, since he managed to match in not only the most competitive of specialties that he was considering, but also, arguably, the most desirable from the standpoint of his professional goals. Yet even after matching, he wasn't sure that he had made the right decision, and mulled removing himself from his obligation to the urology program in order to participate in the main Match for either medicine or surgery. After several days of concentrated lobbying on the part of his friends, who told him he was a bunghole for even considering this course of action, he made his peace with his match, figuring that if worse came to worst, he could always quit after a year and change tracks.

Bob Beatty matched into the equally tough neurosurgery, where he will begin the longest training period of any specialty, a grueling, seven-year ordeal. One other student matched in neurosurgery. It was Andathi, the guy who had clashed so much with Dr. Tomlinson on the Child Psych ward. He's going to a program in the south with a reputation for doing good spinal work, and very little psychotherapy.

Aaron Cosgrove, the man who warned me that I was going to pay a heavy price for working L&D nights, matched into a prestigious neurology program in the midwest. As the year wore on, Aaron and I became closer friends and spent increasing amounts of time together. When I did my Acting Internship I developed a very close relationship with a patient in for her first hospitalization for Ulcerative Colitis. I spent 28 of my 33 days of my AI with her under my care, and when the time came for me to leave (she wasn't going anywhere) she and I sat together and cried for a few minutes while saying goodbye. I felt horrible for leaving her, especially since she hadn't made any real progress. The only consolation I had was that Aaron was taking over my service, so I knew she was going to be cared for by one of the best students in the class.

Overall, our class fared well, I suppose. We had an abnormally high number of people who were trying to match into orthopedics, ER, and radiology — all fields that could have left many people scrambling. However, only four people in the entire class failed to match, and of the forty or so candidates who applied to the three competitive fields above, only *one* was forced to scramble. Lots of people remained in Cincinnati, which is typical for this medical school. An unbelievable number of students — nine in all — matched into the fairly prestigious pediatrics or med-peds programs at Children's Hospital. Two of our students stayed on in the competitive ER program. And one student managed to match in the general surgery program at the University. How big a deal is that? UC students haven't been able to break into the surgery program here for six years. To me, that's probably the most impressive match story of our class — even beating out the guy who matched at UCSF surgery, the one who got into the Duke medicine program, and the one who will be going to the super-competitive pediatrics program in Seattle.

ΩΩΩΩΩΩΩΩΩ

I'm graduating soon, which is a very weird feeling indeed. But I got to go down memory lane the other day. I'm working on the kidney transplant service, which is half-medicine and half-surgery. I've never seen such harmony between these two different professions — there's no hint of the rivalry or condescension that I encountered daily while working both services during my third year. Plus the surgical resident is pretty cute.

Anyway, although I'm taking the course officially as a medicine elective, I asked everyone involved if they didn't mind if I sat in on one of the transplants, since I had never seen one during my surgery clerkship. Nobody objected, and one morning I donned my scrubs, arose at one of those early hours that surgeons regard as late-morning, and headed into the operating room for what probably will be my last time as an observer or participant. I spent my time during the first procedure (where the donor kidney is removed) just hanging back, watching the laparoscopic removal on the television screen. It didn't take much time to remember why I thought surgery was so cool.

Midway through the procedure, the chief of transplant surgery came in, he was going to perform the back-half of the operation and place the kidney in the recipient. "Hey, you here

305

for both of 'em?" he asked.

"Yeah, if it's all right with you," I said.

"Sure. You wanna scrub in?"

"I'd love to."

"Good. We won't get you in too much trouble, I promise."

As I scrubbed in and let the scrub tech gown-and-glove me, I realized that I *knew what I was doing*! At the beginning of my third year, this stuff caused my stomach to quiver with terror. Now it was just *fun* and I was thrilled to be a guest at someone else's table. I wasn't there to get a grade, but rather to witness a miracle, satisfy my curiosity, and contribute to my medical education.

Halfway through the procedure, the surgeon looks at me and says, "Is it Steven?"

"Yeah, that's right."

"Well, Steven, what's that nerve there?"

I was being pimped! At the end of my fourth year! By a guy who knew I was going into medicine! I was tempted to answer by saying that he had pointed to the phrenic nerve. The medical types out there reading this will get the joke. But I didn't want to be rude to my host, the chief of transplant surgery, so I gave the only response I could for a nerve in the pelvis, because I could only remember the name of one.

"Is it the ilioinguinal nerve?" I asked.

"Sarah, do *you* know?" he asked.

"It's the genitofemoral," said the cute resident.

The genitofemoral, indeed. You know what? It didn't matter.

But it was great to review it anyway.